BETWEEN
ZEN AND NOW

A Journey Through The Modern Shamanic Matrix

DR. ASHLEY TOMASINO, DAOM LAC

BETWEEN ZEN AND NOW

Quantity sales special discounts are available on quantity purchases by corporations, associations, and others. For details, contact the publisher at the address above.

Orders by U.S. and Canada trade bookstores and wholesalers. Email info@ BeyondPublishing.net

The Beyond Publishing Speakers Bureau can bring authors to your live event. For more information or to book an event contact the Beyond Publishing Speakers Bureau speak@BeyondPublishing.net

The Author can be reached directly at info@BeyondPublishing.net

Manufactured and printed in the United States of America distributed globally by BeyondPublishing.net

BEYOND
PUBLISHING

New York | Los Angeles | London | Sydney

ISBN Hardcover: 978-1-637922-10-1

ISBN Softcover: 978-1-637922-132

DEDICATION

For Kelly,

May you fly higher than mountaintops,

so high that the wind won't stop you.

"I want to beg you,
As much as I can
To be patient toward
All that is unresolved in your heart
And try to love the questions, themselves,
Like locked rooms and like books
That are written in a very foreign language.

Do not seek the answers,
Which cannot be given to you,
Because you would not be able to live them.

And the point is to live everything.
Live the questions now.
Perhaps you will then gradually,
Without noticing it, live along some distant day
Into the answer."

—Rainer Maria Rilke

TABLE OF CONTENTS

CHAPTER 1

I Will Always Be There

When I was young, I met the most amazing girl who, without knowing it, changed my life in ways that I am still realizing twenty-five years later. What I remember most about her was the feeling of having a true friend. She was someone who really cared about me, not just interested in me because of superficial things, like what bike I had or the type of pens I used in school. She saw me for who I was in the deepest and most soulful way. Kelly was my closest friend while growing up. She was a wise, caring, and loyal friend. We met when we were eight years old from a mutual friend, who was also named Ashley. I remember exactly where I was the first time we met; she was sitting at the kitchen table eating snacks with the other Ashley. I reached out to shake her hand immediately, which, in hindsight, was odd for an eight-year-old girl to do, and I knew intuitively that she would be a very significant person in my life. I felt I knew her right away, even though we had just met.

Whenever I think of her, I am reminded of so many beautiful memories, things she said or did that showed how much she cared for me, the ways she comforted me through life's challenges, and always reminded me that if I ever needed her, I could always call her. I wish I kept the card she gave to me that said, "You can call me whenever you need me." That small gesture of care meant so much to me at the time.

I cared as much for her as she did for me, and this care actually kept my heart open when I wanted to be self-destructive as a way of coping with matters that were taking place in my childhood home. Kelly was a safe friend who loved me unconditionally and always had my back. I am brought back to a memory of sitting together on the grass in front of her house. She said, "Ashley, I want you to know that I will always be there for you. I know how hard it's been for you, and I'm here for you if you need me."

I remember one of the last times we saw each other. We were driving together in her car with a few other friends during our lunch break in high school. Kelly and I hadn't seen each other for a few months because she went to a different school than I did. I remember the moment when the sun was shining beautifully through the window, and it felt like time had stopped. I noticed that she was very peaceful and content in her life, and I could really feel her essence in that moment. I intuitively sensed that she was an old soul who was wise for her age. I told her as she was driving how much I appreciated her and how grateful I was that we could reconnect and grow together as friends. I felt this impulse come through me as I shared this with her that was not just coming from me but from a higher source.

She glanced towards me with a deep eye connection through the rearview mirror in recognition and smiled. She knew something I didn't know but would soon find out. It was an amazing moment to feel so connected again and in such a sweet way. I felt like time had stopped and the world became richer and more beautiful. The light blue and pink colors of the sky during sunset and the softness of the clouds surrounding her silhouette supported this beautiful moment that we shared together. It was so powerful and surreal. I could almost feel as if we were in a movie, and the music on the radio was orchestrating a choreographed experience where we had been transported into another dimension.

That was the last time I saw her alive.

CHAPTER 2

Meeting My Higher Self

When I was 19 years old, I was a sophomore in college at Northern Illinois University or NIU, in Dekalb, Illinois and had just come off the antidepressants I had been self-prescribing two years prior. I was placed on heavy antidepressants starting at nine years old when my parents got divorced. My mom thought it would help me cope, but instead, it made me more depressed. As I came off the drugs, I was beginning to have energetic withdrawals, flashbacks, and intense realizations about my life. I think because I was not living with my mother anymore, I had space to finally start processing all the toxic energy I grew up with. I was in a state of shock and in desperate need of help as the withdrawals started to affect me.

I was so deep down the dark rabbit hole of depression that I had found myself at the foot of the train tracks that passed through Dekalb one evening. I wrote a suicide letter and left it on my desk in my dorm room, where I had hoped my roommate would find it. In desperation, I went to the train tracks, instead. I had a plan to jump in front of a train that evening in April of 2007, only two years after Kelly passed. Before I left the note on my desk, I glanced at her picture on my bulletin board. I felt I couldn't go on with the overwhelming pain and sorrow.

With all the trauma I had experienced growing up, I needed support and help and didn't know where to turn. So, I made the decision to end my life, because I couldn't bear to continue going forward the way things were. I believed I had no reference point to understand what love was, and my struggles with anxiety and depression were so severe that jumping in front of a train seemed like my best and only option.

I walked to the tracks and stood there for a while, crying alone in the brush and trees. Just as I walked to the train tracks to prepare to jump, the conductor came whizzing by with his arms stretched out and yelled through the open window to me, "YOU HAVE SO MUCH TO LIVE FOR!"

I suspect it wasn't the first time he saw someone contemplating life close to a passing train. But what he said made me stop, because his words were so simple—"You have so much to live for."

I repeated it in my mind. *I have so much to live for.* That was the reason I made it there; I felt I had nothing to live for. Words that rang through me like an alarm clock that would never turn off. I stopped and walked away from the tracks to stand against a big oak tree that was nearby. Could it be possible that God had just intervened in my life, through the conductor, and was trying to stop me from this experience?

Even though the conductor yelled this at me, I still got up and managed to muster the courage to walk towards the tracks yet again. I felt this weight holding me back, like my arms were stiff and my legs couldn't move towards the train. *Please, God,* I prayed, *help me. I can't do this any longer. I need help to have peace in my soul.*

I managed to walk towards the tracks, thinking that through death, I would finally have peace. I began to pick up pace to catch the wheel opening, held my breath, and just before I closed my eyes…

Something caught my attention in the sky.

As soon as I looked up, I saw an image of this beautiful woman wearing a white lab coat with long blonde hair, a briefcase in her hand, and standing next to a young girl around the age of three or four years old. There was a man, slightly taller and thin standing behind her with light brown hair. I knew immediately that this woman was me. She was so centered, strong, and at peace within. She was knowledgeable, calm, and serene. But what struck me most was that I could *feel* her from where I stood. Never in my life had I ever had such a strong sense of something outside of myself like this, and I could feel her connecting with me. I could also connect to where she was in life. She had found her center, she had a family of her own, and she was at peace not only in her body, but in her soul as well. I heard a voice say, "This man is your friend for life," referring to the man standing next to the woman, who I imagined was my future life partner.

This was the first time in my life that I had ever felt these energies. I truly did not know peace like what I felt from this woman in my vision. This, I learned later in my year of isolation during a shamanic *dieta*, (I will discuss more in detail later in the book about dietas) was a pivotal and monumental moment where my soul saved me from myself.

I stood back and prayed to God, saying that if He would help me get there, I would do everything in my power to be of service to Him. The ability to see and connect to this image had kept me alive in my body and my soul. I knew that, although I was still deeply struggling, this image was real. The confusion was, *Will I ever get there? Will I ever become her and live in this difficult world as a strong, intelligent, and beautiful woman?* I had to give myself the space to try and see if it would work.

So, I worked towards all I wanted to achieve in the meantime, but I would reference that image to see if I was on track with her.

And when I did lose faith from time to time, when I was hurting, lost connection, or was sick or suffering, that image gave me the strength to work towards a future vision of myself that I prayed to become.

A few weeks prior to the day on the tracks, I had another miraculous experience.

I was on my way to the biology building on campus at NIU in Dekalb on a particularly snowy and cold morning. With my headphones on and listening to Radiohead, I realized the class was canceled and decided to walk back home.

Out of the blue, I heard a woman's voice say very clearly, "Turn around."

Right as I turned around, a car came swerving off the road, towards me. I could feel the little hairs on my neck stand up, and it seemed as though time had stood still. The car was headed right for me.

I then heard this same voice say, "Back up."

Right when I stepped back, the car drove off the road and onto the sidewalk where I had been walking and T-boned a car that was exiting the McDonald's parking lot, right in front of me, where I would have been walking, had I not been alerted by this unseen voice. I stopped in amazement at what had just happened and recalled feeling absolutely still. I felt so shocked by the experience, as if my nervous system didn't connect the dots of what had just occurred.

I wanted to tell everyone. To me, this was God's way of protecting me and helping me by intervening in my life. I always wondered who that was, who that person was whose voice was so clear. Later in my shamanic apprenticeship, I learned that this voice was, in fact, me. It was my higher self. But, how did my higher self know that this was about to happen? I suppose that the divine knowledge and wisdom of our higher selves can recognize forces that may be dangerous and interfere, even if we are not conscious of it.

This logic can, of course, be challenged, such as, *Why wouldn't my angels protect me from accidents, misfortunes, or failures?* These questions are for each of us to contemplate and find the answers to. We all must come to the conclusions for ourselves as to what is real and true for us based on our choices, life experiences, and will for our evolution. Our paths all come with *pruebas,* which are tests that challenge our trust and faith in ourselves, the world, and even God. It was very clear to me while standing on the sidewalk, while listening to "Karma Police" by Radiohead, that I was looked after.

CHAPTER 3

The Initiation

No one ever asks to become a shaman. You are either raised that way due to your cultural circumstances or the experience is thrust upon you; it organically emerges as a life calling from the power of the Spirit. If people knew beforehand what becoming a shaman entailed, they would not even contemplate the task.

I became an acupuncture student at Pacific College of Oriental Medicine in May 2009, just after my Uncle Joe, a mystic and a shaman, had passed away from cancer. He was my hero, someone I admired and looked up to since the moment we met. I played soccer throughout that Spring and summer to try and focus on other things while I grieved his loss.

In October of that year, I mustered the courage to try out for one of Chicago's premier soccer leagues. Earlier that brisk morning, I played in what was the best game of my entire career up to that point. Every pass, every move and decision I made on the field felt so smooth and rich with talent. I decided to play another game, even though I hadn't stretched and was somewhat tired. I had never felt so amazing on the field.

Right before I went to try out for their team, The Windy City Wanderers, I was stopped by the coach, who told me I needed insurance. I paid a small fee, and within minutes, I blew my anterior cruciate ligament or ACL while performing a move called the *cryfe*. It's a move where you drag the soccer ball behind your leg to turn the direction of the ball as you block your opponent. It's a pretty technique to watch and takes some skill to do correctly. I remember my cleats were stuck in the turf when the tear happened, but what was more stuck was my mind. I was confused as to what direction to go, whether I should drag the ball behind me, or trap it and pass in front of me. I had two defenders on me: one to my left and another in front of me, blocking the goal. I couldn't hear any of my teammates, and so I froze. My knee, however, did not. My left knee responded to one part of me going one direction, and another part of me going in the other direction. In a matter of seconds, in what sounded like a gunshot according to the goalkeeper at the opposite end of the field, was not only the end of my knee, but also the person who I thought I was.

This moment was also special, because it marked the five-year anniversary of Kelly's death almost to the exact day. In that five years prior to my ACL tear, I was on a journey of addiction, depression, and perpetual self-abuse. After her death, I self-medicated with all kinds of drugs, as well as being prescribed anti-depressants like Zoloft, Seroquel, and any other SSRI I could find that would keep me from feeling anything. I didn't want to accept that she was gone and there was nothing I could do. After that soccer game, the chains of denial finally broke, and I awoke to the profound realization that if I didn't face the fact that she was gone forever, I would stay in pain, and God only knows what mental state I would have descended into.

It wasn't until my knee injury that I recognized Kelly's death was the trigger for a massive upheaval in my world. It became the initiation that sparked me on the path towards depth and meaning as I searched for a new way to live. As I lay on the ground in pain, I could feel my head break open. There was no way out. I couldn't run away from my pain any longer. Literally.

I couldn't make her alive again, at least not in *this* world. All I could do was surrender and let the feeling of loss fully come over me, the loss that I had been shoving away for so long. All I wanted was for her to be alive again; to hold her and to tell her how much I loved her. There was nothing I could do anymore but lay in a fetal position and cry.

When I say that no one who ever wants to become a shaman would choose that path if they knew what it actually entailed, I say that in the most literal way. The way of the shaman is the most serious path that one can take. My trophies from this path are not shiny objects of gold, rather, they are humility, scars of suffering, and the wounds of soul-breaking pain that the healing journey entails. If anyone would have told me beforehand that this would be the door to walk through, I may have just stayed in my intoxicated state.

The ACL tear seemed like it was God's way of letting me know that there were no more games to be played, and that the world needed me to be grounded in reality. At that time, I came into a relationship with a professor I was studying under. This professor would make a huge impact, not only in my healing journey, but also in my professional development as well.

The moment I truly and finally realized Kelly had passed away and truly accepted it, I happened to be wearing all black that day. I left my classroom because I could feel the tears begin to well up inside and found myself in the fetal position in the hallway crying. I could feel my head split open by the denial I could no longer live with. I was on my hands and knees, feeling almost delirious by the reality and weight of the situation I had been trying to ignore for so many years. I even called Kelly's phone, hoping maybe she'd pick up.

Mary Kay was one of the shamanic acupuncturists and professors at Pacific College of Oriental Medicine who worked out of the Chicago campus back when I attended in 2009. She was a practicing shamanic practitioner with training in Celtic style shamanism and work from the Michael Harner Foundation.

Mary Kay happened to be walking down the hallway when she saw me and approached me and said in her Chicago way, "Get up and follow me to my treatment room, NOW!" she exclaimed.

I made my way to her treatment room down the hall. I laid on her treatment table, and she asked me what had happened. She thought it was something with my knee. I told her as best I could with tears and anxiety about how I had torn my ACL and how I was upset about my friend dying and that I still had not dealt with the grief.

She placed her hands beneath my skull as I laid down on the table and began doing what is called "*a journey*". After a few minutes, she came back around the table and sat down to tell me what she saw while she journeyed. Mary Kay told me that Kelly had a message for me.

This message was that she saw me standing near train tracks and that Kelly said not to follow her. I was shocked by hearing this. How did she know? I didn't tell Mary Kay about the train tracks at the time. She described what Kelly looked like and the reasons she believed Kelly died at such a young age. She told me that experiencing her death was my initiation into shamanism. For the first time in five years, I had a sense of peace about what had happened. I remember changing my whole viewpoint and a feeling sense of clarity coming into my experience. The whole situation suddenly seemed orchestrated for my growth, rather than a traumatic blockage.

This teacher, who was also a shaman, told me this experience of loss would be pivotal in my healing process and would change my life forever. She then told me that she was teaching a shamanic journey class and that I should come. That was the beginning of my journey into shamanic healing with Mary Kay and into the unknown dimension of shamanism.

CHAPTER 4

The Five Questions

After the event at PCOM, I decided to explore moving to San Diego, where my oldest sister, Kim, lived for many years. I recall walking down the street on University Avenue and asking God for a sign as to where I belonged and if it was the right move for me. I closed my eyes and prayed, and all of a sudden, I heard the music playing at one of the restaurants outside. It was Ace of Base playing, "…I saw the sign, and it opened up my eyes, I saw the sign…" Naturally, I decided to move.

After moving from Chicago to San Diego in 2011, I felt the call to journey to Peru for the first time to work with an ayahuasca shaman in the Amazon. One day at my friend Rob's house, I was sitting in his living room in Ocean Beach when a few friends who had just returned from a center in Iquitos called Nihue Rao, appeared, looking very calm and relaxed after their ten-day retreat. They had just returned from their flight and showed up at his house. The moment they arrived, they approached me and looked me deeply in the eyes and one of them said, "Ashley, you need to go to Peru, we were talking about it on the flight, and if I were you, I'd call them and schedule a time to come as soon as possible." Knowing very little about what ayahuasca was,

I decided I should go to the jungle seeing how much pain I was still in and how adamant they were. I was also inspired by how different they felt energetically. The girl was softer and more relaxed than I had ever seen her, and she was someone who I trusted, so when she told me this, I knew it had to be something important. Becoming a real shaman wasn't even the goal. I was still suffering so badly that I was desperate enough to get on a plane and fly to the Amazon for my own personal healing.

The combination of drugs and alcohol, the daily mental suffering, and all the negative energy in my life was killing me from the inside out. By the time I decided to journey to Peru after hearing about ayahuasca from my friends who had just returned, I was already "out the door", so to speak. I could hardly go another day without the weight and suffering I had been carrying. The journey work I had done with Mary Kay was helpful and gave me some relief and clarity, but it was not enough. The pain I felt every day on nearly every conceivable level, is more than I am even able to describe.

I would compare it to imploding on the inside, while my soul was suffocating at the same time. I was unable to sleep, nervous and worried about everything, feeling deep stomach and heart pain, and beset with a perpetual fear that I would never be happy, and that there was no reason to live. On top of all of this, the surgeon who operated on me put screws in my knee that were too large and cut off my hamstring ligaments. This left me nearly handicapped for four years, until I could get insurance to cover the cost of removing them. I couldn't flex my left knee more than 10 degrees without feeling like I wanted to scream.

All of this suffering and more was who I believed Ashley to be. Little did I know that the true Ashley was an entirely different version of the one I saw in the mirror. The version I would discover was the reflection of God, not the reflection of all that darkness and pain. When I looked in the mirror, I saw a sick girl who no one loved. I saw someone I was ashamed of and couldn't live with any longer.

The world was a hard and cumbersome place for me to live in for many, many years and at that point, right before my first journey to Peru, I was ready to give up. So ready, that the Universe tested my faith in a way that was so strong, it would change my path forever, yet again.

Prior to leaving for Peru, I had to attend my internship and complete my hours for the semester credit before I could head off on the journey to South America. I was an intern at a children's hospital in San Diego called Rady Children's Hospital, practicing acupuncture for children with chronic pain syndrome (CRPS) and cancer. I had only a few weeks to wait before my flight left for Peru, and I was preparing for the trip by finishing my clinical internship hours at school. I was still in so much pain and could barely wait to get on the plane to Peru. I counted the days until I could leave.

When I got to work at Rady's one day, my supervisor handed me a chart for a girl who had been randomly placed on our floor when she was supposed to be in out-patient, rather than in-patient treatment. I treated mostly out-patient cases, so I didn't have a ton of exposure to really serious conditions at the time besides cancer like viruses or communicable diseases. So, I took the chart, read over it, and saw she was diagnosed with tuberculosis. I walked to her room and knocked on the door, where there was a little window to peer through. I noticed a plaque outside the door that said I had to wear a face covering because of her condition, so I prepared with a mask and gloves. I saw her facing the veranda out the window below as she stood there very still. When I knocked on the door, I saw she didn't move. So, I knocked again and let myself in.

"Hello, I'm Ashley," I said.

She slowly turned and made eye contact with me. Her eyes were deep, bright blue, and magnetic. I suddenly stopped breathing and focused on her. I stuttered a bit and realized that perhaps she was more than just a patient. This was my intuition; some higher knowledge within me knew something about her was special.

"I'm here to help you; I'm an acupuncturist," I said. "Have you ever had acupuncture?"

While still making eye contact with me, she sat down on the hospital bed. She looked like she was maybe twelve or thirteen. She took a while to answer me, then said, "What is acupuncture anyway?" I explained in a simple way that it was an ancient system of healing that used needles.

She could sense my sadness and pain, I believe. She looked at me and continued questioning what I was doing. During the whole time of our initial conversation, all I could think about was the pain I was in. It was so deep and so raw, eating away at me from all angles that I could hardly talk or breathe. It was as if all I could do was watch myself, like I was outside of my body and I had to watch myself go through the motions. I navigated my way through the conversation as best I could. But instead, she stopped me and started asking her own questions.

Tears rolled down my cheeks, and I hoped she couldn't see. "Dr. Ashley," she said, **"What is the meaning of life?"**

This startled me. It was like a mantra or a command that pulled my soul to the moment. My hands had been working on finding acupuncture points at the time she asked the question. I immediately stopped and looked at her. I contemplated what she had said for a moment and responded, "The meaning of life," I held back my tears, "is to learn and to grow."

"I think so, too," she said.

Even though I didn't feel it in the moment, I had always felt and believed those words. I inherently believed that we, as souls, come here to advance our consciousness, to brighten our light, and to share it with others in the world. I believed in the power of ascension, that the development of oneself through a series of experiences can align us further with what we know about our true selves but have forgotten.

She kept going and calling me deeper into the present moment. Sometimes, when we suffer so much, we forget why we're here and we forget our truth; that there is only the present moment. Suffering is not present; suffering is heavy and dark. It is its own reality, and it sucks you into it, if you are not aware or conscious of the dimension of it. *We must be strong enough not to succumb to suffering's willful power to dispel our light. Holding the light close will deter the ability for darkness or suffering to enter that space, the precious and sacred heart space.*

I believed all these things, but yet I was still suffering so deeply. Then she took a breath, looked at me in the eyes, and said,

"Do you believe in God?"

I paused for a moment, in disbelief at what I was feeling on the inside, almost like someone had reached in and felt my soul and pulled it up, "Uhh..." I stammered. I looked down at the ground, away from her body where I had felt the heat coming from her bones as I placed my hands upon them to do energy work and feel for the points. "Yes, I do." I did believe once, but I couldn't feel, understand, or know what God was anymore. I had lost my faith in a higher power because of the pain I was in.

But I knew that this must be God trying to reach me in some way. When she asked the question, it was like a part of me had stood up and finally remembered what was true for me. I had always been spiritual, religious to some degree, and always a searcher. "Yes," I repeated, "I do believe in God," as if saying it again affirmed it in my bones. It was at that moment that I knew God must be there with me, because something was going on within that room that was beyond my control, and that something was a miracle. God is that lightbulb that goes off when you have that *ah-ha* moment. I was inching my way to that feeling and experience one moment at a time.

I was beginning to wake up and shake off the feeling like I wanted to just die. I had been so focused on this girl that I began to forget my own pain. It was mesmerizing to listen to her and feel her focused on me. I knew she could feel my intentions, and I knew that she wasn't just here to receive acupuncture. She was here for something much more than a treatment from me. *She was there to wake me up.*

Before I could say anything more to her, she asked,

"Do you believe God loves you?"

I felt innocence. I looked down and thought the question: *Do I believe God loves me?* I guess so. I wasn't really sure what God felt towards me or who God even was at that point in my life. I passively believed that God was a man in a white robe with a beard and held some sort of staff, kind of like Santa Claus, but taller and not so fat. If I didn't know for sure that God existed, there was no way I could know that God could love me. That moment, I felt that there was nothing inside of me to love. I felt unlovable, unworthy, and without purpose. How could God love something like that? I had memories of being tormented in high school by my crazy ex-girlfriend's mother, chasing me across the track when I ran track and cross country, with her middle finger in the air screaming 'F-you!' to me, because she was disapproving of my relationship with her daughter. I was that kid in high school who would drive down the street on the way to school and certain people would scream 'Faggot!' to me through my open window. It was heartbreaking. I was told that being gay was wrong, and that I would go to hell for it. I was told that I didn't deserve friends, that I was better off dead, that I was a horrible person for loving my girlfriend. I was told by the adults I knew that the way I loved was wrong. Parents would prevent their kids from spending time with me when they found out I was gay. I felt so sad while growing up. I couldn't understand how the love I felt for her was wrong when inside of me, it felt so pure and real.

I felt that if my friends couldn't love me, how could God? It was confusing for me to establish any real sense of self when the people around me seemed to hate everything I was or stood for. Unfortunately, it was by being in love with a girl when I was in high school and her Catholic family being very disapproving of this, as well as the community I grew up in, that helped to shape my ideas about whether or not God loved me. "God hates you, you deserve to die," her mother would say in response to our coming out about our love for each other. The memory flashed before me about the restraining order they placed on me in order to prevent us from seeing each other. I recalled the time when I was banned from my soccer team because of this restraining order that made it so I was violating it if I went back to soccer practice, since she played on the same team as I did, and of course, I would be within 500 feet of her. I missed out on the opportunity to be a better and more skilled player after I was forced to quit the team. I thought that at school, I could continue playing soccer, but the high school coaches also benched me for a season when they found out. I was shunned, judged, ridiculed, and banned from my club league, because others were unable to accept me. There was no reason for the restraining order. I had done nothing wrong, and the report was full of lies my ex-girlfriend's mother told in order to justify filing it with the police.

I think I was a decent soccer player, and all I wanted was to be a professional, to play on the U.S. Women's National Team. At least, even if I wasn't on the A team in my club leagues, I wanted the opportunity to try and go far with it. Without opportunities at my high school to eventually be recruited to a college league to try out for and play on, my chances were extremely limited. At that point, I had a reputation as this 'faggot-criminal'—or so they called me, that I was doubtful any coach would help me go forward. I was devastated, and with no one to advocate for me, I was alone in the fight for justice and sanity amongst the hate.

Her parents felt that I was entirely to blame for their daughter's decision to go against their mores. We were innocent kids. But I trusted them as my elders, and believed I was unlovable and did not deserve respect for who I was. *They must have been right*, I thought, *they are adults.*

"Yes," I replied, "I believe God loves me." She knew I was lying.

Maybe God loves us enough to intervene when we are about to do something that is so far from our life path that we need something to wake us up and help us remember what we are doing here. Divinity knows no time, but it does know a path, like how a river flows past the rocks that lay upon it. There is a force that keeps us in a space of understanding; we need only look beneath the surface to understand and connect to the current that drives us all. I was disconnected from this current; the current of love.

"Do you believe God has a plan for you?"

Giving the soul direction and remembering our life purpose are one and the same. She had to ask this question. It was only this question that could give me a sense of perspective from the pain I was feeling, even if only for a brief moment, so to get my mind out of the wreckage of the past and remember my soul's mission for having entered this reality in the first place. If God's plan was for me to suffer, I don't think I would call him a God. My suffering was not part of the ultimate divine picture—at least the picture I believed God wanted for me. Suffering is a choice, and in this moment, I could choose to see my life as part of the divine picture, rather than a punishment for having less than what I thought I should. I began to breathe in recognition that perhaps this idea may be true. I felt like there was something bigger than me operating here, and its plan for me, whatever it was, did not end with me in pain.

"Yes" I said with a sense of uncertainty, "I believe God has a plan for me."

She shook her head in agreement, "I believe God has a plan for you, too."

Her final question hit the soft spot, and that was when I knew for sure this was not just a coincidental encounter.

Why her?

Why then?

Why me?

It was the perfect wake-up call for a perfectly lost and confused person such as myself. Prior to this day, I had tried everything to ease the pain I had been feeling. Techniques such as meditation, counseling, working out, acupuncture, and various medications. You name it, I tried it. What made it worse was that I had taken years of pharmaceutical drugs for depression that had only frozen the emotions in my cells, keeping me from experiencing the magnitude of the release that was necessary to finally let go of the grief from having lost my best friend and the stress of growing up in an extremely toxic and dysfunctional household. I was not even in college and was already experiencing multiple nervous breakdowns and thoughts of suicide.

Suicidal ideation is a whole other world of consciousness that takes everyone and anyone it can get its tentacles on. Like an octopus, suicide feeds on its victims and grows with each soul it takes. It brings suffering not only to the victim, but the victim's family, community, and the world. I believe that we emit this consciousness into the ether, the cosmos, and to each other. This little girl was receiving something I had put out, and that something was deep despair.

"What happens when we die?"

I contemplated, "Well," I said, "when we die, it is very similar to being alive, but we do not exist in our physical body." Souls can be stuck in the state of death if there is a trauma or if they are unaware they have passed. But if there is a soul that helps us to the other side, or a trigger that helps us remember our truth, it is like a guide that assists us to stay on our path, even after we have passed away physically. When we die, we don't actually die, we continue, because the journey never ends. To think it just ends is a fabrication of the mind because the mind only knows limitations and distinctions, black and white, up and down. In the spirit world, these essences exist, but they are not concrete. They are essence, which has only the energy of thought.

I had allowed all of my pain to breed darkness within me. I lost my imagination, the part of me that is innocent and connected to the light. In one sense, I already was dead. On the inside, the light was out. It may also have been covered up, but either way, I couldn't see the light until she asked me these questions.

It took me a while to recover from this experience. When I left the hospital room after saying good-bye to her, I went home to my apartment and sat on the couch for what felt like days, trying to understand what just had happened. My mind and heart had been blown open. That was the last time I saw her.

But if that experience wasn't enough to shake me, there was even more to come before my trip to Peru.

CHAPTER 5

You Do This for Everyone Else

Two weeks later, just before I was about to leave for Peru, the tension I felt within began to arise yet again. I found myself sitting on a rock in the company of beach-goers on an afternoon in San Diego. Alone on the rock, I gazed out into the horizon. I felt helpless, out of control, and lost. I was giving up, and I wanted God to take my soul back to wherever I came from.

I wiped the tears from my eyes as five teenagers came towards me. They were all wearing backwards caps, hoodies, and skateboarding shoes. They were about 15 to 18 years old, with that look in their eyes like they wanted to change the world.

"Hi," said one of the boys, "can we ask you some questions?"

"No, I want to be alone," I said. I was resistant to talking with them. I just wanted to be alone with my pain.

"Well, we would like to talk to you," said another one of the boys. They all came closer to me. The one in the green hoodie kneeled down next to me and said, "We'd like to show you some pictures to see what you think. *Please* take a look."

"Fine." I figured it wouldn't hurt. I wiped the snot and tears from my face. My mouth had a frozen frown on it when I looked at them. I noticed it in my reflection on the pair of sunglasses the girl in the group was wearing.

I looked at the pictures. They were held together by a metal ring. The first picture was of a few people walking across the street, much like the Beatles' famous picture on Abbey Road.

"What do you think, what does this remind you of?" asked the girl of the group softly. She looked at me with the sweetest eyes.

"People are walking together on their path. Togetherness, enjoyment."

"Sure," she said, "but what else do you see?" She turned the page to another picture. It was filled of various religious symbols. "Which one do you like?" she asked.

I pointed to the Star of David. It was the symbol that had always attracted me. I began to contemplate why that was. I was someone who often made people uncomfortable with my belief systems, values, and what I stood for. I had cowered and covered my light, so other people would not be uncomfortable. This made me suffer deeply.

She turned the page to a man standing on top of a mountain with his hands in the air, smiling, "What does this mean to you?"

I wasn't exactly sure at the moment. I looked at the picture and drew a blank, but realized that they were giving me clues, clues so that I could remember my truth and to reawaken my soul. When I saw this picture, the woman inside of me sort of stood up.

"I don't know. He seems happy, at peace with life," I said.

She turned the page to another picture. It was of a community of people together holding hands. I put the book of pictures down and looked back at the mountain to take in what was happening.

Two of the kids looked at each other and then back at me. "We'd like to ask you some questions."

It didn't occur to me that perhaps there might be a theme with these questions. They proceeded, very gently and calmly.

"What is the meaning of life?"

I laughed for a moment, "What?" I asked.

"What is the meaning of life?" one of them said.

"You have to be kidding me. I was just ..." I stopped. I remembered the girl in the hospital bed. "The meaning of life," I said, "is to grow, to learn, and to experience."

Where was I? I was starting to come back again to the present moment, remembering weeks prior when I had been even more emotional and upset by life. The kids continued their questions...

"So, do you believe God loves you?"

"Why are you asking me this?" I said bluntly.

"Try and answer the question. Think about it," said the oldest boy.

I answered after a few moments of thinking. "Yes, I believe God loves me."

"Do you believe God has a plan for you?"

I remembered the hospital again. I was charged, the forces around me were thick and sticky, and it was hard for me to breathe. It was like these kids were pulling me out of some existence that I had forgotten, where I was lost and stuck. *Okay*, I thought, *I can remember, but where are you? Where is God?* I could only question. This questioning brought me closer and closer to the other side. I was reaching up and out, "Um, yes, I believe God has a plan for me."

Ashley, wake up! It was like someone grabbing my shoulders and shaking me uncontrollably back and forth. Wake up and remember who you are, this is the only salvation you can achieve.

I remembered my friends grabbing my shoulders when we hung out in the forest. Alicia shaking me and looking me deep in the eyes saying, "Wake up, Ashley, we love you." I was so numb.

I began to cry. I had felt this way for so long that I had forgotten what it was like to feel deep joy that was not distorted by superficiality or fake-ness to please others.

They kept asking their questions.

"What happens when people commit suicide?"

How did they know? I looked around at all the other people on the beach, swimming and surfing in the water near us. People playing with their children, eating lunch, living their lives. I thought I fit in there, that no one would notice.

I was a little startled by this question. "People commit suicide," I had to think about it for a moment, "because they are stuck in the same reality as they were when they died in their last life. They are still in that frame of consciousness, the consciousness of taking one's own life, a state of trauma, perhaps, or self-hatred. They try to escape, but they cannot, because you cannot run from your experiences if they are within you. In order to release them, you must feel them, transform them, and let them go. When people commit suicide, they are shutting down their light from the experience of God's love, the love of the Universe and flow of all things."

"If you commit suicide, you cannot move further, because this is like school. You will be stuck in the same space that you were in anyway, but this time in spirit, where the work needs to be done in the physical on the physical plane of Earth," said one of them.

"I can't take the pain any longer. I want to give up."

"Don't give up, *there's so much more to live for.* There is joy to experience, you just have to be open to it. Recognize that it's there for you to have and that you are worthy, with or without the job, the title, the car, the money, or the fame. You are perfect just as you are, and you are perfectly deserving of the same joy that any of us experience. All you have to do is ask for what you need. You are not alone," one of them said.

They stood up, and they began to put their backpacks on and prepared to leave, "We have to go now. God loves you, Ashley. Remember that God has a plan for you."

As they began to walk away, I turned to them and said, "Why did you stop for me? Out of all these people, why me?"

The oldest of them turned and said, "Because, you do this for everyone else..."

I looked back down at the sand beneath my feet, and they were gone by the time I said goodbye.

Guides show themselves in the physical realm at times, whether discretely or in more obvious terms. They'll give you signs that they are present, but they never interfere with your process, nor obstruct the flow of what you are meant to experience without your permission. Just as with other relationships in life, each guide you meet serves a different purpose. It may be to help you through a transitional phase, or to help you become more compassionate. Whatever the mission, contract, and purpose of the relationship with your guide, you will learn and grow. My experience with the girl in the hospital and the kids on the beach are examples of how I know that guides are real.

CHAPTER 6

Welcome to the Jungle

I arrived at the Los Angeles airport after a bus ride from San Diego. Exhausted, I found my way to a breakfast place to sit and relax before I headed on the plane to Iquitos, Peru. I was excited and nervous. It was my first time ever leaving the country alone, and I had no idea what I was about to get myself into. I knew very little about ayahuasca, except that it was an Amazonian plant medicine, and I was not entirely aware how much I would be drinking upon arrival to the center. To be honest, I wasn't even sure at all what I was doing, only that I had to be there and surrender everything I was carrying in my soul.

I stood in line for my connecting flight to Texas when I had second thoughts. What was I doing here? Do I really need to go all the way to Peru to learn how to heal myself? I closed my eyes and began to pray under my breath, "God, please give me a sign if I'm meant to go to Peru."

I closed my eyes and looked down. When I opened them, I saw a boy in front of me with a pink backpack on that had white hearts and said, "I love you, Ashley."

Surely, I felt this was a sign.

I arrived in Iquitos with my oversized luggage on my back that I borrowed from my then boyfriend, and with my two feet standing on Peruvian soil for the first time, I knew immediately that I was in unchartered spiritual territory. I was in a territory that I could not have dreamt. Prior to having made the decision to go on this adventure, I spoke to my mother over the phone about it. She insisted that I should not go and yelled at me that God didn't exist and that it would be dangerous for me to be in the jungle all alone. I'm glad I didn't listen to her, because all of the things she said, like how I needed to protect myself from tarantulas, jaguars, and other predators, were never an issue.

A sign with the name *Allison* was waving in line as I approached the exit terminal at the Iquitos airport; a short dark-skinned man named Marco was smiling and holding it out for me to read.

"Are you Allison?" he asked in his Peruvian accent.

"No, Ashley."

"Oh, okay, same thing. Where you from?"

"The United States, California."

"Yeah, you the one I am waiting for."

I hopped in his *mototaxi*, and for the first time, I saw the epic and mysterious Amazon Jungle. It took over an hour from the airport until we finally arrived in a small village called Llanchama where the center was. My eyes were wide open. I had never before seen stray dogs, people selling food on the streets, or babies on motorcycles speeding past us nearly driving into oncoming traffic. I saw three people sitting on one motorcycle driving down the unpaved road. I saw vendors selling coconuts and cheap bottles of soda. I smelled the exhaust from the trucks and fumes from the factories. I was in a type of heaven I didn't know existed. It was a radical experience, and I had not even made it to the center yet.

When I arrived, I met a few people who had been there for some time already. Some were ready to leave; others were planning a longer stay. The first person who greeted me was a doctor who ran the center. He explained a few of the basics about the center regarding the layout and where I would be staying, but overall, I still didn't really know what I was doing or where I was, only that I had to be there.

I brought a lot of baggage — mental, emotional, and spiritual —to the center, and I knew I needed help letting go of so many things from my past. At first, I saw a few *tambos*, the small jungle huts where people sleep and stay for a time, and the *maloca* in the middle of the center, the place where the ceremonies are held. I had my own bed in a quiet area, except when the birds would squawk in the morning as loud as possible.

I met with the master shaman, Ricardo Amaringo, to state my intentions and explain why I was there. Ricardo is the shaman who founded Nihue Rao Centro Espiritual. He is a native Peruvian who initially started his training by performing what is called a *dieta*, a long period of isolation and spiritual training out in the jungle for over a year. He was also an apprentice to Guillermo Arevalo, a well-known *curandero* who also leads ayahuasca ceremonies in the Amazon. Upon first meeting Ricardo, I felt a sense of respect that I had not felt before and was humbled by his powerful presence. I could tell he was a compassionate, hardworking man who genuinely cared about helping the people who arrived at his center. Through meeting him, I was inspired to learn and explore this medicine work that was so new to me.

I was not sure why they needed to know all of my biographical information, but I felt safe and explained what I wanted to gain from the experience. I was told that before any ayahuasca would be served, I had to drink the *vomitivo* to clear my stomach of any toxins. The *vomitivo* is a brew of onions and a pulp from the tree called *oje* that causes you to vomit when you drink it. Once you get some of it down, you're likely to start projectile vomiting. It is my least favorite drink! I wondered when I would encounter Kelly in any of my ceremonies.

The first night of drinking medicine, I arrived at the maloca, which was in the center of Nihue Rao's property. A maloca is a large hut where people can gather for ceremonies. I found my mat and patiently awaited my time to come up in front of Ricardo and drink the brew. I had no idea what ayahuasca was even up to the point that I was sitting in the maloca about to drink. As I approached the brew, I could sense the auspiciousness, especially with the bugs in the forest and the night sky as it fell upon us. Everyone was quiet as they sat with anticipation of what their night would bring. I said to one of the ceremony assistants who served the cup to me, "go big or go home" when they asked me how much I wanted. They poured me quite a large glass, and I could see the ceremony assistant smirking as I drank.

Within about an hour, the affect kicked in. I was thrust into a world that was completely unknown, and I could feel something like an asthma attack coming. I was afraid, and the fear caused me to cry helplessly out for my mother. I had to control myself, so as not to actually scream out in front of everyone for my mother—that would have been embarrassing! Instead, I called out for Jose, the assistant, which was a powerful moment for me, because I was processing the loss of my beloved Uncle Joe, who had passed away only two years prior.

My Uncle Joe was a shaman and a mystic who I admired and loved dearly. He was the person who I called out for whenever I needed help, and especially when my parents divorced. I was suddenly thrown into a memory of sitting in my grandmother's kitchen the first time I met him and remembered his presence in my life. He sat at the table and told me, "Ashley, all there is, is love." He also told me as he looked down at my penny loafers with pennies in them, "you deserve dimes." He took out some dimes from his wallet and put them in my shoes.

At this point in the ceremony, Jose had arrived in front of my mat, and I looked at his face and saw a lion. I was in the midst of a whirlwind of emotions, confusion, sadness, grief, and despair. He blew mapacho smoke (a type of tobacco used in the Amazon that is stronger than regular cigarettes) over my body, and I suddenly felt better. Before he did that, I heard the medicine say, "Breathe, Ashley."

I felt calm and at peace and sat back on my mat and journeyed into another dimension within. I could hear Ricardo singing with the other shamans in the background during my journey and felt like I was in the right place.

I also began to remember what was in my heart, and I was brought back to Kelly. The tears and the crying were so immense that I couldn't hold back any longer, like a dam that had exploded. I had held it in for so many years because the antidepressants had blocked my senses and ability to process the grief. There was no holding back, and even if I tried to stop crying, I couldn't. It was coming out with all the strength that I had held it in.

I was brought back to her funeral. I remember I stood over her coffin and tried to cry. I wanted to, but nothing would come out. I felt ashamed that I was so numb from the antidepressants that I almost had to fake it to show she mattered to me in front of her friends and family. Even when I gave her eulogy, nothing came. I remember standing behind the podium in front of at least 100 people, giving the speech about how much I cared about her and who she was to me. It felt so surreal and my mind was unable to grasp what happened. Perhaps it was shock, but I think I needed the environment necessary to really let it out. As the dam exploded in the maloca, I couldn't stop crying for days. Overwhelmingly, the tears were more than I could have imagined I could produce. It was more than just the pain of her death—it was also the guilt that I didn't save her.

I remembered the last conversations we had and hearing her say, "No one would care if I died." The guilt began to show itself, and there was no one I could say sorry to except myself.

Because of how much I drank, I was still in the mareacion and tripping for two whole days afterwards. I sat in the hammocks the next morning that were hanging outside the maloca and watched lions in the trees and faces of their spirit everywhere.

I was reminded of how much my mother shamed me growing up for being a Leo. She would snicker at me, "Oh, you're such a Leo." She hated my grandmother, because she was also a Leo, and therefore, I should be ashamed of who I am intrinsically.

The breakthrough was that I began to learn to love myself on a very deep level through this vision of a Leo that came to me. The lion in my courses with Mary Kay was my spirit animal. I had been doing a soul retrieval by recognizing this power and reclaiming it. For so many years, I was shamed for my birthday, by my own mother, who had total control over this if anyone does. This was the start of my stepping back into who I naturally am and was.

The next night, I drank again and wondered when I would meet Kelly in my ceremonies.

And then, suddenly, in one ceremony, she appeared. I saw her standing next to her grave site, looking down at it in trepidation. I was glad to see her finally, but then she said, "Ashley, I'm afraid to go there." I felt as if she was projecting that fear because of some false belief system she carried in herself. I said to her, "Kelly, wherever you go, I'll go there and find you and bring you back. You won't ever be alone, no matter where you go. I'll always be there to help you, so there's no reason to be afraid."

And just like that, the scene changed. I could feel the grass beneath my feet, and the sun shining in the distance. I embraced her in a hug and held her body close to mine. I could feel her bones and her spirit, caressing her hair and feeling the beat of her heart, as if she was alive again.

As I held her, I could feel that she suddenly evaporated into the light, and her body became the light. I stood there feeling the immense power and energy from this love. I knew she went home to a better place, and I felt a deep sense of peace inside, finally.

CHAPTER 7

Meeting God

The future enters into us,
in order to transform itself in us,
long before it happens.

-Rainer Maria Rilke

During the time I stayed at the center, I could feel more of myself coming back, pieces of my soul returning and integrating into my body. I began to feel lighter, and that the things that had bothered me for so long were starting to be cleared.

But towards the end of my two-week stay, I started to feel stifled again by some overwhelming emotions that were coming and going. And even though I was making progress, something still felt stuck inside of my bones and my body. Something was still bothering me at a very deep level. I wanted to move forward, but the weight of memory that I could not let go of still seemed to haunt me.

On the night of my last ceremony, I decided to contemplate how I would receive the medicine. I was feeling triggered again, and I had a small argument with another guest at the center. I remember before walking out to the *maloca*, I was lying on my hammock and began to pray. I prayed to God to take me away from this place of pain that I had been in for so long. Why did I need to suffer so much? I went to my mat in the *maloca* and sat there with all parts of me ready to surrender to the medicine.

It was my turn to walk up to the mat where the ceremony assistant served the medicine. This time, I was going to access a deeper place within, and I had an open my heart to all the possibilities that could potentially meet me. I wanted peace; that was my only intention.

I went back to my mat, relaxed into the space, and began to hear the *icaros*[1] from a distance. The master shaman started pulling things out from within me and around me with his words, a language that I did not totally understand. I did not understand, but the songs felt so raw and real to me; I could feel them clearing my soul and cleaning the debris from years of hurtful thoughts and things I had experienced. My visions began to open up, and I saw a dark figure in a room built like a *dojo* with Japanese paintings and bamboo floors. It appeared almost like the room in *The Matrix*, with Neo and Morpheus having their first simulated fight. I became Neo for a moment, and then I began fighting my own ego — it was in the shape of a man in dark clothes trying to kill me. I wanted to fight back, but then, I remembered that love transforms all darkness. So, I gave my ego a hug.

I started praying for help to my angels and guides. With the next breath, my vision began to open, and I immediately saw a gap in the floor where I had been standing in this alternate universe that then transformed to a vision of spinning knives. These knives were layered in what seemed like endless rows, where they were rotating quickly

---

1 Icaros are the songs a shaman sings that are medicinal, not just to sound pretty or to sing for fun but they connect with the melody of their plant medicines which can help the patient. Icaros are chanted in various languages and are practiced as a form of treatment in places like the Amazon and other shamanic traditions.

and in different directions. I felt the urge to jump through with my ego, knowing that when I landed, anything that was not real or true in me would be demolished. I jumped through, hoping to find a space where I could land and be safe from this strong force of darkness that was opposing me.

I jumped into the abyss of knives with the intent that when I was done with this journey, I would be lighter and freer from whatever held me back. I could literally feel the blades run along my skin and crush my bones, melting memories off my body like a knife cutting through butter. I could hear metal scraping across itself as I fell through several of these rows of blades that cut across my body and soul, clearing anything I did not need for a new phase of my life that I felt myself entering. I finally crashed to the ground and laid there in disbelief. I had disassociated from my physical form and appeared in another world completely, a spiritual world.

After looking around to new my surroundings, I saw a ground made of musical glass squares lined next to each other, all with different checkered colors. As I stepped onto the glass, they made beautiful music like piano keys. Looking down, I peered through the glass at a directionless universe. I had no idea what was forward or backward, north or south. All I could see were stars beneath my feet. To the left and right of me were galaxies pulsating next to each other, as if they were connected to an infinite fabric of time.

I looked up and saw a shorter man, like an elf standing before me, wearing a velvet blue suit and shiny loafers with dimes in them. I smiled and noticed he had information for me. He began explaining what I was doing there.

Apparently, I was lost, and this being knew it. He explained in a clear, but strange voice that had a melodic quality, like music, that he wanted me to know I was in a safe place.

"Where am I?" I asked.

"You are in another world, Ashley. One where you can dream and imagine the world into being, a world where all of your wishes are here for you to manifest. Please come with me; I have lots to show you," said the elf.

I followed him through a door that appeared suddenly. When he opened the door, I saw rows of leaders from all over the world sitting inside of government-like building. These leaders were the presidents and vice presidents of the galaxies, not just of our planet, Earth. I was led down along a red carpet to the seats that were designated for Earth and sat amongst the leaders. I looked around to the various faces; some were not human at all, and it reminded me of *Star Wars*! I began to feel excited, because I had heard and did not know of this before, but I was in the presence of the Galactic Federation. They did not communicate via words; they communicated through telepathy. Because I was so excited and could not stop chattering in my mind, I called a lot of attention to myself.

Various leaders in the cosmic assembly turned to me, because I was so disruptive with my thoughts. I could hear one of them say to me, "In order to stay centered, you need to clear yourself of the ego, because it is the ego that destroys the possibility to have telepathic communication between people, as it is of a heavier frequency." The frequency of thought is one emitted through a very fine frequency, and I suddenly realized the whole congress was communicating telepathically. Most were communicating through openings in their crown chakra and heart chakra.

I left the federation and walked out of the room, through the same door I had entered. As soon as I closed it, I looked up to find a massive white staircase before me. I was weighed down by the pain from my family, the pain I had caused others, and the pain I had carried throughout the years. Back in my physical body at the ceremony, I put my hands together and could feel the force between my palms. I began to pray.

"God, please forgive me!" I cried, as I could see and feel the pain I caused my family. I could see the pain I had caused friends and ex-lovers. I continued asking for forgiveness over and over again. I began to see the connections between myself and others fade away, like bodies falling off me and into an abyss of nothingness. One after the other, they got further and further away from me as I prayed. I began to feel lighter as the weight of the pain I had held onto began to lift. As more fell off of me, I could suddenly see more clearly how this weight had affected my soul. I had a new perspective that allowed me to realize the beauty of my connections with others, even if they had not been perfect, and that the relationships had not lived up to what I had hoped and imagined they would be.

For some reason, I got the sense that all relationships are made of souls brought together until we can fully forgive one another and feel the magic that the transformation of such binds allows us to feel. It felt as if I would not see the true magic between myself and others unless I was truly able to let go. It took great courage to ask for forgiveness, because it meant that I had to open my heart to those who had hurt me, and to truly loving myself as well, even though I had caused others pain. What a scary thought!

I turned back to the staircase and saw the first few steps. I reached and crawled on the first step, knowing I had to ascend, and that this was the way to the light. It felt like I was carrying pounds and pounds of bricks as I began to ascend the staircase. "Please, forgive me," I cried out. The load got still lighter off my back, and I was able to crawl to the second step. I turned again and saw even more people I had hurt behind me.

"Please forgive me!" I said louder. I'm sure people around me could hear in the ceremony. It was like a chord had snapped from my back to these people and experiences. Slowly, they fell behind me, like I had undone a tightrope. I could suddenly breathe.

I was able to walk up more and more steps until I made it to the top. "Thank God," I said to myself. I continued to feel a state of gratitude and thankfulness for the weight being lifted from my soul. The light began to flicker first like a little beam in the distance, and then, it grew to a circumference around my body. Images became clearer, bright, and glowing gold with white glistening sparkles of a fabric made into railings ascending above the airy clouds.

With a sense of serenity, I basked in the knowingness that I had made it to my destination, wherever that was. I had no idea what the details were, but this deep sense of *knowing* came over me, and I could not resist looking around at the vastness of this new infinite landscape. I was expanded, connected, and open.

I saw ahead there were rows of faces of all the gods lined up next to each other, emanating outwards above a white podium that stood in the distance. It was tall, maybe eight feet high, with the brightest light shining at the top, hovering above. I could barely make eye contact, because the light was so bright, so it was difficult to focus on the specific details of this tower. However, I knew it was something conscious, as it was *observing me just as I was observing it*. Formless, faceless, it was so bright that I had to look away. I saw Buddha, Jesus, and all the Hindu gods. I saw all of the ones I've loved, cherished, and honored in the rows beyond the limits of what my mind could comprehend. I was in awe.

I saw Krishna, Shakti, Ganesh, some god with blue skin and a pierced tongue. I saw the Egyptian gods, pharaohs, princes, queens, and kings in their light. They were all one with Christ consciousness, connected to source, but yet defined by their own unique blueprint and self-realized with the same understanding that they were part of unconditional love. And as they manifested before me, all I could do was ask…

"Um, can I come in?"

"Hmmm…" said the bright white light. I could hear this voice as clear as day. I could hear it just as clear as I can hear the music playing on my laptop as I write this now. *The being* thought for a second, and I could feel a playfulness (and I refer to the being as 'he', because the voice had a lower pitch than what I would imagine a woman would have.)

He was smiling. With a mallet in his hand, he hit the podium.

"Accepted!" he exclaimed.

I was confused. "Me?! But…I'm not a doctor, I don't have a lot of money, I'm not perfect…"

I began to make more excuses. I wondered if I had died, since I heard that the light above a staircase is where you enter the gates of heaven.

"Did I die?"

"Yes." Said the being. "You had a spiritual death."

I looked back at my body on the mat, lying there motionless.

I realized how happy I was, and had not felt this in a long time. "Can I see my life? Like, in the movies, where it's slow motion and I can view all the events?" I asked.

"Sure." The being laughed. I looked away and saw a sin cosine wave near me made of bright lights. In between the troughs were images of moments where I experienced life. I saw my birth; I saw my life's moments where I experienced pain and sorrow. I saw all the love I had and the holidays. I saw the Christmases where I would open gifts, or when my father would hold me over his shoulder as a baby and play clair de lune on the piano. I saw the days when I ran track and cross country, my first kiss, my first crush, my first pet dog, Teddy, and all the fun we had. My heart had bust wide open. It was a glorious, gorgeous display of life.

The being then stepped off the podium and suddenly transformed into what appeared to be a human. He reached his hands to me gently and said, "My dear, I am not human."

"Then, what are you?" I asked. I could feel so much warmth and love emanate from this being. I knew he was here because I had to fully accept it into my consciousness.

"You humans believe I am a human because I am a reflection of your consciousness. But I am not a human. I simply AM. I am from another dimension."

"What dimension?"

"The dimension of *love*. This is where I am from," he explained.

I could see as he explained this dimension, as if it were another planet! People in this world were harmonious, kind, and peaceful. Everything moved with grace and ease.

"Would you like to know how I created you?" he asked. Suddenly, I could see the faint qualities of a human, like a younger, healthy man wearing a white gown, holding himself with dignity, respect, and deep inner peace.

"How?" I replied eagerly. "How did you create me!?"

"With just a thought, Ashley."

I could barely contain myself. "Wha-What was the thought?!"

"The thought was *love*."

He continued to explain. "There are many versions of love, there are many versions of our reality as we perceive it based on our belief systems. The thought for you, was that you would be created in the perfect image of what love was to me. You were created in my image."

Then, he asked if I wanted a hug.

"Yes, yes I want a hug." Yes, I wanted a hug from God! Duh!

When he hugged me, I felt a recalibration from every cell of my being, as if I was lit up with a complete sense of deep, universal knowing. I felt completely in bliss, so warm and forgiven. I felt accepted for who I was and in a deep state of relaxation.

He pulled back, and it was *me*.

He transformed into what was the perfect version of me, with blonde hair and a beautiful blue dress on. She was smiling and happy. I could see her blue eyes and light skin. She said, "I created you in my image." Her voice was so clear, soft, and beautiful, like silk flowing from her heart and out her mouth, even though we spoke telepathically.

"You see," she said, "love takes on many forms. In life, there are many colors and shades in the spectrum." She pointed away to a few TVs with various images, "There is pain and suffering, babies being born, war and cruel acts of hatred, love and lovers, nature, beauty, peace…all of that is love. All of that that you see in these TVs are versions of various aspects of love and what it means to be part of the world of consciousness, awareness, and all that you can experience."

"So, then, what is the *meaning* of life?" I asked.

She laughed. "Wow, everyone asks that question!"

"The meaning of life, Ashley, is to have an experience! You see, look at all of those experiences in the TVs. People can choose to have these experiences, and it's all okay. Whatever they wish to feel or experience is up to them. It is all available, depending on what station they choose to tune into."

I could feel this being did not have judgment about any of these things. She was completely detached and removed from the nature of anything happening. She simply had compassion, understanding, and respect for the experiences each person chose to have.

"Pain and suffering are a human condition. It is a choice to maintain the pain within one's field and live in it, although some disagree. However, I still love you."

"God, please, please forgive me for all I've done. I've been such an asshole to all of these people..." Before I could continue, God stopped me.

"I already have. I have forgiven you before you did anything. It is **you** who does not forgive yourself."

I sat there in contemplation and relief. I recalled all of the times I had heard people say out of anger that they would never forgive me for something I had done in the past. I realized that a truly loving person embodies this feeling of forgiveness, because forgiveness is love.

"You are my child, and I created you in my image exactly as you are. You are perfect in my eyes," She said with love.

"So, if you're God. Can I ask you for some things in this life?"

"Well, sure! You can ask me anything."

"God, I would really like to help others heal, and for there to be more healing in my family and the world. I would also really love my own family."

She showed me all the people who would benefit from a new age of healing, and I saw the happiness in my family and in my world. I was delighted to see the details and the joy emanating from each soul I witnessed in front of me.

I went back to the place I met God, near the podium, and sat down next to this being.

"Okay, God, wow. So, can I have one more thing in this lifetime?"

She smiled brightly at me. "Sure, Ashley, anything you would like."

I took a deep breath, looked at her in the eyes and said, "I would like to have an amazing career, one where I can affect thousands of people in a really positive and impactful way."

She snapped her fingers, and suddenly, I was on stage in front of thousands of people. I was actually looking at myself in the future from behind myself. As the perception changes, like in a video game, I was able to look at myself from a lot of different angles. I observed this woman from behind the stage and watched her as she confidently and courageously talked to all of these people about topics that I did not know anything about at that time. She was referring back to a large screen behind her that had a diagram with something scientific.

She was talking about an evolution of consciousness, but her intention was unique. She was using the speech to transform her audience, as if they were experiencing a healing. As she spoke to the crowd, at first, they looked like monsters, all with scary faces and evil eyes. But as she continued and spoke from her heart, without a doubt in her mind, she was able to speak to the hearts of these people and turn them from monsters into beautiful children, eagerly listening to stories of bright beginnings and possibilities for their dreams to come true. Waves of light washed over these beings before her, and they were magnetized one by one by the sincerity of her speech.

I returned to the mat in my awareness and felt a sense of hope for my future, unlike any other time in my life before. For the first time, I felt a true sense that my dreams could come true.

CHAPTER 8

La Madre, Mother Ayahuasca

Opening to the world of plant medicine implies a journey into the shamanic matrix of life. The shamanic matrix is the world of shamanism that allows us to connect to an altered state where we can navigate the dimensions beyond our mind. When I refer to the shamanic matrix, what I see is an alternate universe that is present as a mirror reflection of our current reality. When people connect to ayahuasca, what they're looking for is the ability to transcend the mind and go into that matrix. In my courses, I teach people how to enter that space and navigate it. But that matrix is something that the plants and the shamans understand deeply and subconsciously.

It is an encounter with the collective consciousness of vegetative life and the natural world. And the highest expression of this plant consciousness is the Mother, ayahuasca. It was only after I entered my year apprenticeship that in the ninth month I finally met her face-to-face.

It felt like I was her daughter, and she was the mother I never had. She knew everything about me and accepted me for all that I was. In the presence of ayahuasca, I came to understand that my journey to wholeness was releasing the old version of myself, a version that I had constructed as I related to my own mother in this lifetime. She embraced me with warmth, tenderness, and the care I desperately needed as a child. I came to understand that my journey as an *ayahuasquero*₁ meant I had to heal my relationship with my mother, so I could transform into a medicine carrier, without the imprint of trauma from my past. When *la madre* ayahuasca held me in her arms, it was a moment of deep peace and healing that I had been aching for my entire life. I realized in that moment that my own mother needed this herself, and her mother, and for that matter, all of the children in the world.

As I allowed this new experience to enter my space, I felt layers of suffering shed like old skin off a snake. The softness and strength of her was like a big tree in the forest. It was a unique connection that opened my heart and helped me feel the real Ashley within.

Embracing *la madre* means that you become open to her love and teachings. Even if you are suffering or if there is resistance or blockage — the deeper point is to just try and open yourself to her loving presence. When the intention is honest, no space exists for pain on the soul level.

La madre is not just with us when we drink. The mother is always with us. Even if we are blocked or afraid, her consciousness is present. I had come to believe through past experiences that if I did something wrong, the love I needed would punish me by abandoning me emotionally or physically. That was just a belief, though. The truth is, because the plants don't have human-like agendas or egos, nor embody our human character traits and flaws, they are much like witnesses in our journeys and don't punish.

Unlike what most *curanderos* I have met think, I do not believe in punishment by the plants. If we do something out of integrity,

1   An ayahuascero is a healer that uses ayahuasca.

there may be a natural cause and effect, but at no time did I ever feel *la madre* was attacking me. I think that is a religious view that has been ingrained in much of the way people think about reactions to unpleasant events when encountering the power of ayahuasca.

The understanding that comes from the plants is profound. These qualities are what *dieting* allows us to feel. When we work with plants, the wisdom of compassion gets transferred to us in ways we may not have ever known before. And so, to perform a *dieta* means that we are stepping into a sacred and contained space, so we are uninterrupted by outside forces to receive the direct transmission from these sentient beings in plant form.

It is said that as we learn from the plants, they, too, learn from us: it is a synchronistic relationship between plant and human intelligence. The sharing of our own energy with the plants and our intimate engagement with their world allows for their consciousness to grow as well. The imprint from our relationship with the plants helps fuels their own healing, thus helping them grow and help us in return.

When I first met the medicine, I often felt like I couldn't breathe when I was under the effect. But I never felt that ayahuasca was to blame. Rather, the medicine was helping me to see how in my own life I felt suffocated and stressed. I grew up with asthma. I had to take an inhaler to sports events and keep it with me whenever I got stressed or went out with friends. When I first started working with *la madre*, I had many breathing problems and panic attacks that were, most likely, due to stored traumas and memories of panic from childhood. My mother would often yell at me so strongly that I remember having difficultly breathing. In general, I always seemed to feel like the air around me was thick and that I was constantly gasping for air.

The first time I ever had an asthma attack, it was actually me pretending I had one. I was a cross country runner in high school and junior high, and I was running in a cross-country race. Typically, I came in second or third at worst, but this one race I was falling really far behind to the last group of runners. My body felt incredibly heavy, and I couldn't understand why I couldn't be at the head of the pack. Usually, I was ahead, but on this particular day, I was having trouble just moving my legs. I was so ashamed for my seeming failure that I got on the ground and pretended to wheeze.

My coach, Mrs. Rosenfield, came running over to me. She was a younger coach with blonde hair and was attentive and caring towards me. I don't remember what happened next, but the doctor who examined me ran a few tests and discovered I did, in fact, have asthma.

I was told that I had "stress-induced" asthma and that whenever I played sports, I had to have my inhaler with me. I never told my mother about the fact that I faked the wheezing attack, but when I took the inhaler, I immediately felt like I could breathe so much deeper and relax. The albuterol helped me in future track events, eventually assisting me make it all the way to state finals for the 4x400 and 800-meter dash. Every time I took the inhaler, I had this edge and could speed past my opponents. I remember preparing for a race in the state finals, sitting on the bleachers near my teammates' parents, who watched me inhale the albuterol, take a few caffeine pills, and get hyped up for the next race.

I saw the look on a woman's face. She was concerned and disappointed. She knew a little about my life, as her daughter and I were friends. I felt like all the parents knew about me and how hard things were for me. A few of the other parents during my childhood let me know they were there for me if I needed them. I could feel concern from the adults around me, so after that race, I realized I needed to face the fact that I was abusing the inhaler and had to deal with the fatigue.

During my *year dieta* at Nihue Rao, I recall sitting in a ceremony and suddenly seeing that moment in the race when Ms. Rosenfield came to me. My intention that night had been to clear the alcoholism from my family, and so, I entered the ceremony space without knowing where or how deep that would take me. The next scene, once the effect came on, was of myself on the ground and Ms. Rosenfield standing next to me to check if I was alright. I had completely forgotten about her for almost twenty years until then. This opened more memories where I was shown her perspective of me and her concern observing me from a distance. The medicine can open repressed memories that help to unravel what may be at the root of our problems and aid in the discovery of the deep traumas that may be hidden in our psyche.

I was ready to face this sad moment when I had outright lied; faked an injury because I didn't want to own up to how much help I didn't even know that I really needed. I was proud of myself for the speeches I gave on running, friends I had made, and winning races, but I was not well.

During the scene where I kneeled on the grass in Ms. Rosenfield's presence, I felt the medicine show me the depth of the sickness in my soul from alcohol in my family. Although I was not a drinker, having alcoholics in the family affects not just the drinker, but also the others who they are relating to as well. In programs like Adult Children of Alcoholics, as I understand it, the entire family is affected by the alcoholic. Some members may be enablers, while others may join the problem. The alcohol was not just from my immediate family, but my ancestors and distant relatives as well.

When I connected to this deep feeling in my soul, it felt like an endless dark cave filled with yellow pus and dark energies, what we call *mawayoshin* in Shipibo terminology.

Mawayoshin energies are like ghosts of the past that have no consciousness in the light. It's a dull, dusty kind of energy with some level of will attached to it, which makes it like a ghost.

When they say that alcohol is spirits, I believe alcohol contains *mawayoshin* and perhaps *yoshinbaum* as well, but that is just my theory. Yoshinbaum is a term to describe spirits with much more will and intent who are dark and have an evil quality to them.

I noticed within my soul that I had accumulated not only my own sick energy by not caring for myself, but also the sicknesses that had been passed down to me from my ancestors on the soul level.

After working with *la madre*, I found that we may never be fully aware of our own pain and ancestral trauma, and that our intentions are opportunities to dive deeper into the unknown within. We will eventually be shown what is available to energetically heal, as well as room to process, so we can recover and come back into centeredness again.

I had to take a lot of time after this ceremony to be with what I was shown. I was humbled by the care and magnitude of the messages from that journey. I realized that not only do we make illness real by pretending it's there, but the power of our words and how we can call in problems unconsciously.

Many of my ceremonies for the first few years I worked with the medicine were basically hours of gasping for air or asthma attacks on some level. Panic attacks were frequent for me as well. I grew up in a state of panic and insecurity about my life, so working with the vast and infinite world of shamanism was overwhelming, to say the least. When entering any space, we have a sense of the dimensions around us, where the walls are, where the bathroom is, how to find the exit. In shamanic space, the worlds are infinitely vast with no firm boundaries to place our hand on and identify as we journey. *La madre* teaches us to always come back to the heart as the center and compass to discover the particular direction we need to go. Because my heart was broken, my world was chaotic, and I couldn't trust my caretakers, and entering ceremony was sometimes terrifying.

Luckily, I was blessed with facilitators who could understand some of what I was going through, because of their own histories with depression and stress. I found myself particularly bonded to one of the doctors at the center where I apprenticed at. He changed my life completely, because it was the first time I felt someone could not only see me, but treated me like I was worthy; like a real friend who wanted me to succeed. This friend helped me to forgive my own mother and focus on the beautiful person within. He allowed me the room to feel pride for being a Leo woman, for being an acupuncturist, and for other qualities that had been covered up by the sadness and shame I carried.

La madre has a way of bringing people together and helping them learn lessons, find love, grow, and open to new relationships.

It should be said that not all work with *la madre* is so arduous and challenging. Sometimes, the most profound healing with *la madre* occurs in sitting after ceremony in a candle-lit *maloca*, speaking with someone you care about and learning more about their life. Sometimes, the most powerful healing is allowing *la madre* to open your voice, so you can sing for your friends or those who are suffering. Or maybe laughing with friends and enjoying the moment. These experiences put everything into perspective because you are embracing the moment as it is while you are healing.

When I met *la madre*, I projected onto her all of my traumas and ideas I had about what it meant to work with a force I didn't know.

After finding myself in deeper spaces of healing around my own mother, I was able to see *la madre* with clarity, and let me tell you, it was such a sweet and beautiful experience.

CHAPTER 9

More Healing with Ayahuasca

A yahuasca shamanism is a spiritual practice of connecting to the wisdom of vegetative consciousness. The brew, a combined mixture of the *chacruna* leaf and the *banisteriopsis capii* vine, when taken orally, produces an intense psychoactive experience for the individual. When working with ayahuasca, it is important to understand that there is a way to connect with higher spiritual states and to begin the process of healing. Just knowing there is a way can bring a sense of deep relief. And from there, you can begin the important work of healing with that knowledge acting as a supportive and loving force.

Through conscious communication with spirit, a shaman acts as a portal to support the integration of divine consciousness with the physical world. Traditionally, in various indigenous communities, the role of the shaman was to maintain the overall health of the community. The shaman served as a leader, priest, doctor, seer, mediator, and psychologist for the tribe. The shaman helped with decision-making, offered guidance, and ministered advice in any dire situation. Using specific talismans and magic, the shaman would even perform exorcisms when necessary, working with strong energetic forces to restore health within the people, the land, or in the water.

Today, in developed western economies, people are using pharmaceutical drugs to numb, rather than really deal with their problems. People are experiencing intense levels of anxiety, depression, cancer, and other illnesses at an alarming rate. It is no wonder that there is a growing population of psychedelic users and plant medicine practitioners these days. I have seen people come to my office for years, ever since I began my practice, who are deeply ill and not recovering from their traumas and pain. People are looking for answers, hope, and support. People are looking for safety and community.

We are looking for God.

And for each of us, this is a unique and different entity. But the one thing that remains true about our relationship to God is that we are innocent in the eyes of this Being. This innocence is our most powerful state, and it is in our innocence that helps us to connect to our humility. In being humble, we are able to journey much more effortlessly and efficiently through the realms of spiritual existence. When this happens, we stop searching, and we start *being*.

There is no need to feel lack, because we are inherently whole by the very nature of recognizing what the truth is, which is that all is fine and that everything is perfect. But the problem rests in the fact that our nervous systems have become so strained; we have been traumatized by life, we have inherited the pain-bodies of our ancestors, afflicted by the thoughts in our heads and by the habits we have cultivated and learned through our immersion into society, and deeply hurt from our families and our unique life circumstances.

What this world desperately needs is a real awakening to our divine truth.

We cannot assume that by simply putting a pill in our mouth, or even sitting in an ayahuasca ceremony and letting visions come to us, that all our problems will go away. I have seen countless people with many years of experience with the ayahuasca brew who have had no visions or deep spiritual insights. They simply did not understand that you must *actively engage with* and work within the worlds of shamanism to achieve these kinds of insights. You can't be a passive observer in the healing process.

When the *mareacion*, or the peak of the psychedelic affect is felt, many people I have spoken to assume they are experiencing the shamanic world, because they see colors and shapes, moving objects and pictures appearing in their vision. However, the real shamanic space requires a journey beyond the view of simply an observer with your eyes closed. I teach this in my courses. The path to engaging with the real shamanic space is to go beyond the visions, lights, and colors. This is done when you engage in what is called a "journey". The journey begins with a conscious decision to engage with a memory; it can be a safe and neutral memory from your lifetime, or it can be a traumatic one.

After that, I teach my students to find a portal or a location where there is a space to either ascend or descend into the matrix of the world of shamanism. Typically, we are taught to find a tree and descend through its roots to what is called the underworld. The underworld is generally the first level of worlds we can travel in, so that we may face our darkness and make allies with animal or plant spirit guides that can help us throughout the duration of our journey. By doing this, the experience goes a little deeper, and the journeyer enters a much more profound altered state, while experiencing another level of empowerment, because they are actively engaging in the process —

rather than simply being a passive observer — of moving through the matrix with intent.

Oddly enough, many people I've spoken to, people who worked with the medicine, even up to 500 to 1,000 ceremonies, said they did not have deep visions. They reported that they only saw colors and lights or senses from their feelings. They had these experiences because they were not accessing the shamanic matrix. I was surprised and wondered if they knew how to truly engage with ayahuasca in the way I had been trained to do through the core shamanic way of journeying, as taught in Mary Kay's teachings, back in Chicago. Although Mary Kay was not a practicing *ayahuasquero*, the tools and systems of journeying she taught me were very supportive in understanding how to navigate the ethereal realms of consciousness within. After applying these tools, I felt I had a secret weapon, a way to engage with that world from a centered and empowered place. I appreciated the core shamanic way, because I was able to learn how to journey at any time in the day or night without psychedelics, simply by drumming or tapping on my desk.

I remember sitting in one of my classes at Pacific College of Oriental Medicine as I was taking an herbology and formula making test. One of the questions on the test was, "What two herbs would you give your patient for a prescription in their oatmeal who has headaches? I didn't know the answer, so I gently tapped on my desk and closed my eyes to "do a journey", as Mary Kay would tell us to do if we didn't know something. So, I descended into the lower world and fell into a little boy's body who was just about to scoop up his oatmeal in his spoon when I looked down and saw the herbs he zhi ma and he tao ren. These two herbs are used for headaches and can be added to our meals. The two herbs are sesame seeds and walnuts! I came out of the journey and wrote the answers down and got it right!

This was the surest way I could begin applying my journey techniques to everyday life and while working with *madre* ayahuasca. I figured that if I could access those realms without the medicine, surely, I could with it, too. These practices helped me to navigate the spiritual dimension in a more empowered and conscious way.

Sure, we can surrender to the experience and lose our need to control our reality. Sure, we can let go of the responsibilities of the day and let the drug infuse us with the oneness that the flow of life brings. But what if there was more to it than just opening our mouths and swallowing the medicine?

I began to understand the importance of the tools that are being described in this book after meeting more and more ayahuasca drinkers who had little to no deep shamanic experiences like I did. They would say they saw colors and lights, but what I was seeing was like I had been living in a completely different world, where I could actually feel, see, and interact with my spirit guides, as if they were right there in front of me. I assumed that my practices with the drum and journeying *without* medicine was what prepared me for a much more deep and captivating experience. It didn't matter how much medicine I drank; I was able to work with the tools of journeying with the drum to enter portals and take myself to alternate realities and back safely.

I believe that we are all capable of tapping into this shamanic matrix. Some of us are born shamans, and have a natural ability to see, hear, and sense other worlds; we have tendencies and alignments within that have allowed for a natural capacity to understand what shamans around the world know to be true. Other people have to learn these tools and discover after practice. But you don't have to wear fancy garments or elaborate jewelry, nor smoke tobacco, nor play your drum at a bonfire to be called a shaman. In fact, most shamans I know don't dress up at all, unless they're in ceremony. Most shamans I know don't even call themselves shamans.

By connecting to a deeper level of reality with shamanic practices, we can transcend the ego and allow God to flow through us. The loss of ego determines our experience and magnitude of the mystical moments we encounter. The more we release the ego, the more we see the beauty and connectedness of the Universe; and yet, at the same time, we face some more challenging realities that may arise the deeper we go into this space. It seems our ego pops up when we deny or resist what is appearing as truth and may not have the tools to fully process.

Death of the ego is the hallmark of the breakthrough we strive to accomplish, and that marks the true ascension of our soul; but it is what we are also naturally afraid of as well. Death of the ego can be the death of our entire world, depending on how much we have allowed it to infiltrate our belief systems and consciousness. What if death was just a transition and that transition could be an opening into another beautiful dimension representing the evolution of our consciousness—something not to be feared, but to be embraced with dignity, humility, and respect for all we have learned?

After the experience of seeing God in my vision of 2012, I became very interested in continuing my path with ayahuasca. I found myself connecting to more ceremonies and different styles of practices. The medicine has a way of helping us to recall repressed memories. The brain is not the only place that energies and past experiences are stored. I learned in college while I was studying biomedical science that we store memories in our gut as well, otherwise known as our solar plexus. This, I would later learn, would be the primary place for me to focus my healing. It also seemed to be the general place where people store their emotions and what the shamans of the Amazon refer to as *ocha*. Ocha is also known as being the same as our faults, our sins, and all of the bad energies that compose feelings like guilt, shame, and fear. The excess energy stored in the solar plexus region blocks us and clouds our energy field, preventing us from having the space to receive and emit love from God and other people. This is what ayahuasca can help us clean and heal.

CHAPTER 10

Crying Into My Drum

In 2009, Mary Kay from Chicago became my shamanic teacher after the incident where I was laying on the ground crying and having a massive breakdown. I attended her courses, which ranged from journeying both into the underworld and towards the upper world, finding guides, learning about how to clear intrusions, extraction work, clearing dark energies, and doing soul retrieval. Our group consisted of myself, Daniel, who was another student at PCOM (Pacific College of Oriental Medicine), David, and Kerri. We met every Sunday for four hours or so and practiced journeying for ourselves and each other. Each week, Mary Kay had a different course objective in mind. Sometimes, we would share chocolate or other food together and then explore the realms within.

For the first time in my life, I felt that I had a skill that I could properly apply that made my spiritual world make sense. I also learned that I was very good at this type of shamanic work, and that I had a lot of natural gifts in this area. I was particularly impressed by the uniqueness of these shamanic practices, like our journeys to the middle world or astral projection techniques, in which we would encounter places around the block to see what they were like in the 1800s, distorting the space-time continuum.

Mary Kay would drum while we would lay back with eye masks on and undertake a journey. These experiences would then become the foundational blocks that formed my sense of confidence with working with ayahuasca. I realized that these inner navigational tools allowed me the capacity to transcend aspects of my mind, because the drum softened the voices in my head; the mental chatter that had always seemed to orchestrate my world.

Many years later, when I was living in San Diego, I realized, still without my acupuncture license yet and needing to work while in school, I would apply what I learned from these courses with Mary Kay and from my ceremonies in the jungle to create a company called The Advocates. This business was a shamanic business where I helped people with problems such as soul loss, intrusions, and spiritual attack. I found an office that was inexpensive to rent by the hour, and I had my drum and some tobacco from Peru that I would smoke.

I remembered my old business partner from my earlier company, Awaken Therapeutics, once told me that if you want to be successful, you have to create your own system. He also told me that I should do what other people are doing, but do it better. This was some of the best advice anyone has ever given me.

So, I did just that.

I developed a system of helping people that involved a sequence of three drumming sessions in an hour, during which I would journey and gather information for the client. The session began with tobacco being blown on their shoulders, top of their heads, and across their chest. This process involved my own style of healing that also incorporated a special process called *tobacco blessings*.

These tobacco blessings allowed me to bless my patient, making them feel comfortable with me, and it also allowed me to diagnose their energy while looking at them from the perspective of a shaman as I blew the tobacco smoke from my pipe onto their shoulders, heart, head, and feet. The tobacco blessing was also a way for me to diagnose the patient, because I would see how their energy changed when I blew the smoke on them. Just like in Chinese medicine when we take pulses, I would take the pulse of the patient after blowing smoke on them, to see how their energy shifted, or even if they were uncomfortable with me being closer to their body, in order to reach the tops of their head or shoulders.

Then, they would lay down while I drummed for about an hour, breaking between journeys to tell them about what I saw and what I did. The drum became an instrument for shifting energies while they thought about their problems, which caused a charge in the energy field around them. To my surprise, I was very good at drumming, and I found both a pace and a rhythm that allowed them to safely go into a trance. I was able to explore their space, share honestly and with kindness about what I saw, and help them have new tools to take home, so they could make the changes they needed in their lives.

This was so powerful that I began teaching others how to do this. Then, I offered workshops, apprenticeships, retreats, and other classes that helped people go deeper into their process. I learned a lot about business, and running one taught me how to become a more responsible member of the community.

But this didn't become an overnight success by any means. It took me two years of making maybe $200 a month or so, borrowing money just for the $125 a month rent, and praying for help just to make a change. In the beginning, I really had to trust my drum and the journey work I was blessed with. I thought, *How could I have gone through so much and it be worth nothing?* I had to keep focused on the goal, which was to help as many people as possible, and share the message of shamanic hope.

I recalled one of my shamanic teachers had said, "Your drum doesn't become your drum until you cry into it." One day, I went to my office after not passing my acupuncture licensing board for the second time and sat on one of the chairs in my treatment room. At that point, I was deeply in debt, making less money than a teenage babysitter does each month, and unsure of where my next paycheck would ever come from. I had to take the boards for the third time and borrow money from anyone who was generous enough to offer it. I was scared and humiliated, afraid that I would be stuck in this situation forever.

I remembered a conversation I had with my ex-boyfriend, "You know, Ashley, I don't want to date someone so sad like you." And it got me thinking about what truly made me happy.

I remembered how happy I was when taking Mary Kay's class.

I cried into my drum and sat on the chair in my office, feeling defeated and wondering how I would ever be able to share my good medicine and support myself, without having to make my way back to Chicago with my tail between my legs, in debt, desperate, and alone.

When I cried into my drum, it was like a miracle, because all of a sudden, I realized that I could teach what I knew. I didn't even realize that I knew so much until I started teaching, but I felt like I could just share the basics about drumming and tobacco blessings. So, I went online and created a one-month workshop that met every weekend on Sunday, just like Mary Kay taught, including having people share chocolate. At first, I only had one person signed up. Then, my roommate said she'd come. I figured, *Alright, I have two people, plus me, now I just need two more*. I eventually signed up two other people and made a whopping $1,200 for this one-month program.

It turned out to be a great experience, because it allowed me the space to engage in the process of integration. I was integrating all the medicines I was given from my time in ceremony and throughout my shamanic journey work in Chicago. I realized I knew a lot more than I realized!

Then, I taught another course and signed up nine people! And then, I taught another and signed up 12 people!

I surrendered to my own medicine. That is how it happened. I took one giant leap into believing in myself and suddenly, I was my own master. It was incredible.

Crying into my drum was a form of deep surrender, letting go to the magic and the mystery of the Universe and honoring the divine gifts within me. At the time, I was battling with some unseen forces from colleagues who were also in the ayahuasca community. One of them told me to my face that I didn't deserve to be a shaman, and that she was doubtful I could ever be of service to anyone. Frankly, I didn't understand how she could be so rude, but I took it as an opportunity to show her what I was made of and that she didn't have a leg to stand on when it came to the strength of my knowledge and the wisdom of the medicine I was blessed with. I kept going, despite her doubts, bad mouthing me, shaming me, and accusing me of things that I'd rather not even say. She was something like an enemy, and I could feel her whenever I worked. But I kept going. I kept helping people and minding my own business. People were drastically getting better in my office. People were coming in with 20-year problems that I was able to help clear with only one session.

If I listened to her, I would never have helped so many people and in such a deep and meaningful way. I'm glad my drum came through. It was a powerful and potent time to be alive. It was a powerful time to step into my power and own what I knew. I look back and see that she was helpful, essentially because without that type of opposing force, who knows if I would have cared so much to prove her wrong.

CHAPTER 11

Transcending the Teacher

In shamanism, it's important to find a teacher who will guide you as you take your journey. The teacher may appear when you least expect it, which oftentimes is the best way, as it is the Universe presenting a guide when you are ready for the next phase of your journey. The phrase, "When the student is ready, the teacher appears" is often effortless and guided by synchronicity.

However, there comes a time when the path asks the student to grow without the support of the teacher, and this becomes a unique initiation; for the student to discover a new faith in their own abilities. Not all journeys in which we move on from a particular teacher are smooth, but when you are ready, you will know, because you will see your teacher in a different light, or perhaps on a plane that is equal to yourself.

The best way to truly know is when your soul alerts you that you simply don't need them anymore to show you the way, because they have already helped you find an independence that propels you forward. This can be true in any relationship because all beings are teachers in their own right. Once we have learned the lesson, these karmic bonds that pulled us together can clear, which allows for the space to grow and transcend the dynamic that brought you together in the first place.

I've had mentors who, in the past, were more like parents, playing roles that felt almost like they were my mother or father. At the time, I needed this to reflect an aspect of my healing experience. Once I healed these parts, I was able to embody those energies within, and the role the teacher played as a parent wasn't necessary any longer. If you are looking for a teacher, one who guides you on the path of shamanism, there are some core qualities you should look for within this person, so you know whether they are appropriate or not.

You may find that these qualities in a mentor are some great qualities to look for in other partnerships and characteristics to refine within yourself. The characteristics that a mentor has will allow for more room for growth within yourself. A good way to recognize whether the mentor is right for you is simply to observe how you feel after you work together. Do you feel more conscious, empowered, cared for, and happy? Not all these feelings are necessary at one time, but they are important.

You can probably imagine what to look for when you want to spot out the qualities that would make a master someone to not work with. These red flags often come with the simple yet blatant feeling that you just don't feel empowered around them.

Some obvious qualities are those that make you feel like your boundaries are violated, or when you say no, and the teacher doesn't listen or respect that. The teacher may have an agenda and push their own desires upon you. These negative qualities exist in the spiritual and shamanic community and can often be disguised, because if you're suffering and need help, sometimes, it's easiest to take what is there, and discernment isn't as strong as it normally would be.

I have had experiences in the Amazon where I was taken advantage of during a time when I was very vulnerable and alone. Luckily, I escaped and was relatively unharmed, but there was a man who tried to convince me he was a shaman and could help me when I was unable to sleep. It turned out that he stole money from me by selling me these "magic potions" which were nothing at all, instead causing me to projectile vomit for hours. The experiences I've had in Iquitos were typically not the best, only because I was not prepared, didn't realize how much help I needed to protect myself, and was too trusting. After the shaman tried to help me with banking and translation, I realized he was stealing money from me at the ATM when I wasn't looking and lying about costs of things. Since I didn't speak Spanish very well, I didn't notice until I looked at a few receipts and did the math on my own. This was the first time in Peru that I had money stolen and dealt with a shaman who made me physically—and subsequently, psychologically—ill. This shaman wasn't my teacher in the sense that I was training with him, but I'll give him the credit that he taught me a lot about how people can be and that I needed to be extremely careful, especially when coming out of a *dieta*.

Luckily, I haven't had too many experiences with shamans who were evil or dark. I would say it is rare to find people practicing what is called *brujeria*—black magic or sorcery—because *brujeria* leads to the one practicing becoming sick, themselves. *Brujeria* is the practice of stealing energy through dark magic and violating the space of another. Someone who practices *brujeria* is a *brujo* (masculine) or *bruja* (feminine). These are common terms in the ayahuasca world, because from what I've seen, there is also a lot of superstition. People who practice shamanism are striving towards purity with their practices, to avoid falling into these dark ways of sorcery and magic. A shaman who works in the light will always leave you feeling better and more connected to divinity. A shaman who works in with dark energies will leave you feeling sick—perhaps on multiple levels, confused, and running in loops in your reality; meaning, that you feel like you are repeating the same karmic patterns over and over again.

At some point, everyone must grow and experience the journey without their training wheels, because that is where the practice of trusting yourself and having faith in your medicine happens. What are some ways to know you're ready to leave your teacher? Perhaps you simply graduated from a formal course and the course is now over. Or perhaps you realized you were given everything possible from this person and you're naturally ready to let go; there's nothing more to do with them and nothing more you want. There are certain circumstances in shamanic relationships where once the line of appropriateness has been crossed, the chances of traumatizing a student are severe, which is why you want to be extremely careful with who you work with in medicine and especially psychedelic work.

It can be dangerous to stay in unhealthy mentorship relationships. Because ayahuasca shamanism has no ethical board or advisory guidelines, it's possible that the incidence of abuse or trauma and inappropriate behaviors go unnoticed or are touted to be part of your "lesson". At no point in time should you feel disempowered, less than, controlled, fearful to leave, or manipulated. These are times when you must be strong enough to be your own best teacher and walk away and become your own master.

CHAPTER 12

Becoming Your Own Master

I often see my clients searching for a teacher, someone to show them the way to whatever it is they are searching for. If I ever sense a client is looking up to me too much and it seems unhealthy, I gently remind them that I'm not better than them and encourage them to connect with their own power. The sense of being led by a master in ceremony is important because you want to feel like the leader has control over the space. If you're in ceremony and you know that they have overcome what you're working on, it helps you to feel safe; but ultimately, you want the leader to be strong enough in their own sense of power to let you rise to your own self-mastery.

The mastery I'm talking about is the *mastery over your own medicine.* Your medicine is the connection to what heals your soul. When you have mastery of your medicine, you understand it intimately. You sense it, you know it's yours, and that it is there for you to embody and share with others. A true master never steals this from you, nor do they block it. Rather, they help you to embody it within yourself, without feeling threatened.

I remember sitting in a ceremony in Peru at Nihue Rao, purging something from high school. A deep, painful, dark liquid was pouring out of my mouth into the bucket as Ricardo was singing his *icaros* to me. I recall intuitively hearing this voice saying, "*Master the pathogen.*"

I didn't understand exactly what that meant at the time. Master the pathogen? I thought, *What pathogen?* After doing some investigation, I realized that my pathogen wasn't necessarily a virus or bacteria per se, but a spiritual disease. My spiritual disease was once that of depression, despair, and emotional anguish, related to some core traumas in my ancestry. I came to learn more about this through many months of meditation practice, journaling, singing, and sitting in isolation with the plants to unravel and discover what was deep within that caused so much suffering. How could I possibly master this when the pathogen was so entangled in my very existence, when my essence was mixed in with the very energies that I wanted to purge?

Instead of being consumed by what I wanted purge, I had to release, piece by piece, the very remnants of what was not Ashley. It was a process of diving into my subconscious mind with ayahuasca and my master plant teachers, in order to unveil what was true, beyond the realities I had created with my mind.

The first step to being a master of my pathogen was simple, yet so excruciatingly hard: to take full responsibility for my healing. That didn't mean that I took responsibility for what others said or did around me that caused me to grow ill, but to be so vigorously honest about my circumstances that I didn't make it about anyone or anything else. That seemed to be the only way to hone in on the energies that gave my power away and pushed me into victimhood. It's hard to admit that, but the more I pointed the blame at others for my sickness, it seemed the more disempowered I felt. If I gave the problems over to others who didn't know how to fix it, I would be left without the *icaros* to match the disease. When the shaman learns to sing, they find the melody from the master plants to meet the sickness's frequency. At the same time, it was important in my process to understand that there were people who were rightfully to blame and for me to experience what it felt like to feel honored for the feelings I had around various abuses and traumas due to the treatments by others.

Then, they meet the melody with words, to adjust the way the sickness needs to be handled, whether in the body, mind, or spirit of the individual.

I remember when I learned how to play the drum, at some point, I realized that my drum was teaching *me* how to play. I was learning how to be a "drum rider", a person who plays the drum and then rides the drum's medicine through the core shamanic journeying practices and tradition. Over time, I felt like I was becoming a drumming master, because I was becoming more and more integrated with the wisdom of the drum and learning how to navigate its power.

Just like a horse rider learns how to master riding their animal, a shaman must learn how to master orchestrating the power of their medicine in ceremony with their voice and clear intention. Mastery doesn't just pertain to the shamanic arts. Mastery means that you are fully connected with your craft and know how to work with the incongruences, challenges, and darkness to find your center and the harmony within all things. The master maintains humility, grace, and strength and has overcome the difficulties related to their practice.

To become a master, you must go through a core sequences of events. These events are sickness, initiation, healing, learning, dark night of the soul, recovery, and then, finally — mastery. These cycles that one must go through to achieve mastery are the essential tests to the path of true healing. In the beginning, there is a problem, one that ordinary methods cannot alleviate. The initial problem may also be an event that suddenly changes your entire life, one that puts you "on your knees", so to speak, like the experiences I had in the first few chapters.

When this happens, the person has one of two choices: to continue doing what they were doing before—in my case, it would have been to continue with self-medication and alcohol—or to try something new— to surrender to the process that is opening before you.

When you don't feel like you can ever go back to old ways, no matter how hard you try, that is when you have reached an opportunity for initiation, and ultimately, the humility and grace that follows when you truly surrender to the process.

The initiation is a step in a different direction. You have initiated a new beginning, filled with uncertainty and unknown factors, unlike what you have ever known before. It's an exciting time to unravel what is inside; elements with your soul that you never knew were there; spiritual gifts and spiritual muscles to flex for a new task that your mind could never have conceived before. I remember when I saw myself above the train tracks in Dekalb. I never knew the feeling I had could even be possible when looking at myself in the future, this feeling of peace and power that was centered in such feminine strength. It was beyond my comprehension at the time. An initiation allows us to go places and feel things that are radically new. It's brought to us from a divine orchestration of events or intervention that will inevitably propel us forward towards a new era of living.

Healing after initiation makes sense to me. If birth, itself, is an initiation, healing from the journey through the womb to the hospital bed is necessary. Movement through these channels can be traumatizing and disorienting, to say the least. When healing happens, it's to bring us back to ourselves, into our bodies and taking a deep breath, not just with our lungs, but with our souls. That ideal intention to reach towards after an initiation event is to allow for the energies to set and integrate. The initiation changes us. It helps us to shed old skins and become someone new. The healing helps us to relax into it. When we heal, we let the world calm down and be restful as the intensity of the initiation births us anew.

I suppose learning could be placed anywhere in the cycle, as it can happen at any given moment. We learn throughout the entire process of mastery. We learn so we can move to the next phase of the cycle and not repeat old lessons.

One of my favorite movies that follows this theme is *The Spiritual Warrior*, based upon a book by Dan Millman. In the film, Dan meets his teacher, who works as a mechanic in a car repair shop. When he meets him, he's impressed by his spiritual knowledge. Dan soon finds himself being unwillingly initiated after he breaks his leg. He then has the decision of whether or not he will surrender and learn with what his teacher has to offer. He makes the choice, and then, he begins the true process of healing and learning.

He goes through a series of tests with his teacher that help him to get in touch with the magical essence in life, all the while challenging his mind and ego. The master teacher has special gifts that Dan is intrigued by, and so, he changes his ways of living, because of his curiosity with his teacher's power. Through this experience, he inevitably learns how to be truer to himself and develops a centeredness, which helps him to step back into the gymnastics arena and win his competition. The mind-over-matter practices help him step into his role as his own personal master once he realizes what his teacher has been training him to do all along.

When I began the process of recovery after what I believed to be my dark night of the soul, which arguably, I could say most of my life was prior to finding the medicine, I began to really heal. It's almost like there was a smoothing out. The dark wasn't so dark, and neither was the light so bright. I found that people began to be more relaxed and relatable towards me. I could sleep again, which was a big sign, as I couldn't sleep well for so long, and I was beginning to find good fortune and luck again. I realized I was recovering from the profound affects that occurred throughout this journey, just like I would feel after any challenging experience. Recovery from this process looked something like: lots of rest, good food, exercise, and being much gentler with myself. When you're in recovery, you know you've made it, because you neither feel the extremes of fear, nor the extremes of arrogance. You're calm and relaxed about who you are, without feeling like you need to prove anything. Once you're there, you're basically at mastery.

Humility is the key to mastery. Humility will sustain the practice, because it is an energy that operates with the powerful yet gentle force of God; a force that propels individuals forward, to offer their gifts to the world with the intent to be of true service.

CHAPTER 13

The Only Path to Wisdom

What if I told you that the only path to true wisdom was through making mistakes, the point where you grow into the version of yourself that carries true knowledge and humility? Would you believe me? I certainly was surprised when one of the maestros1 I worked with told me this. He said, "You gain wisdom through mistakes, so don't be so hard on yourself." I didn't understand this at first, because I was raised to believe that I had to be perfect, and that if I made mistakes or acted in a way that made my mother upset, I was physically reprehended, demeaned, or punished in some regard. Instead of learning how to safely grow from a mistake, I learned to be afraid of them, often walking around the house with a sense of tension and fear that I would be treated horribly if I made one. I was always walking on eggshells. I simply didn't know that mistakes are part of being a young girl learning about the world.

We live in a culture where people are hyper-focused on whether they are doing the right or proper thing; and if you do not abide by that unwritten rule of our culture, you may face the intense ramifications of feeling like you are some kind of social outcast. This pressure

---

1   A maestro(a) is another term for shaman but typically implies that they work in an ayahuasca ceremony as a facilitator that directs the ceremony.

was seen for what it was when I was in my *tambo* in the Amazon, because while alone in the jungle, if I made a mistake, there was no one to attack me for it. I began to hear a loving voice gently correct me, instead. I had to keep reminding myself that the plants do not punish. Why would they? They aren't affected by what we do as a human would experience; they don't take things personally like we do. I think that by learning and making these adjustments in life through the view of a loving parent who does not punish, we can learn much more, and the lessons are held in a sacred way, rather than with fear.

The path to wisdom is a spontaneous path of living and adjusting when necessary. The learning becomes part of life, itself, and through continual integration, we embody the teachings we have accumulated over time.

I met a very wise *curandero* named Michael after I closed my year *dieta* with Ricardo. He was a referral from a former friend who saw that I needed guidance to return to so-called normal living. Upon speaking to him, I felt like he was reachable, sincere, and had a lot of experience. What I liked about him more than the knowledge he shared was his ability to be an ally during a time that I really needed it. Through the course of a year working with him, I noticed that the work was gradual. There was no forcing of information, no demands, no pushing me to do or think like him, and no shaming if I made mistakes (and I made plenty). He created a space for my integration in such a way that was unique to his practice and adjusted to what I needed. At the time, I felt very disconnected from my previous community of healers in the lineage I was trained in, but through working with him, I could feel the hope for a new community, which reminded me of what I valued most in shamanism: which is the feeling that we are part of something bigger than ourselves — *a community.*

The wisdom path is actually quite simple. The mind is what makes us think it needs to be complicated and abstract. Although the path contains intricacies and strands of information that are complex, as nature is complex, the wisdom path always sees what is true for us in the moment. For me, the kindest, simplest, and most moderate things always bring peace and truth.

CHAPTER 14

Pruebas

I was born with certain undeveloped spiritual or psychic abilities. These natural gifts became apparent to me as I grew older, but when I was young, I couldn't understand why I was so different from my peers. I was able to see ghosts at a very young age, to astral project, and at times, I was even able to predict the future. I had special gifts that made me hyper-sensitive to the outside world and at the same time extremely scared, often leading to difficulty sleeping, because I could feel things in the house I grew up in—like ghosts and spirits— and I didn't understand why I had such extreme sensitivities.

Our ancestors may have passed, but oftentimes, their spirits are still with us in many ways. Whether it is through their wisdom that has been passed to us, or even their wounding that we have received in our own genetic make-up — there are many possibilities of how we engage with our ancestral past. I know now that my gifts came from own ancestral lineage.

But it wasn't until I began my year *dieta* that I began to notice that some parts of my experience were not directly from me or my own life. There is no way to really know, I suppose, but I do believe that our ancestors can indirectly live on through us. To heal our ancestors and carry on their power, it first requires a sense of awareness and to become conscious that there are elements in our healing journey that are not our own; they are familial or ancestral wounding that we carry within us.

In shamanism—and particularly with ayahuasca work—I've learned that the specifics of ancestral wounding is not always what the spirits are trying to convey to us. Sometimes, we receive this information in metaphors, emotions, and intuitions. We don't have to know the specifics of every detail. The medicine will depict our ancestral wounding based upon its relevance and how we can best understand it for the purpose of healing.

I believe what we are shown regarding our family and ancestral wounding ultimately teaches us about forgiveness, social construction, and at the same time, the destructive power of long-held guilt and pain that has been passed down through the generations. Somehow, I pieced together that these powerful emotions and traces of the past can be transmitted through lifetimes, and we can, with the help of ayahuasca, learn about our genetic past and grow from it.

All tests, like healing our genetic past, are meant to support the new definition of character that we set out to distinguish when recreating our boundaries in the process of healing. When making a declaration to the Universe, it's essentially setting an intention of what we are to become, and to set the tone for how we will carry ourselves in the course of the journey. In becoming a shaman, I had to face many tests, and sometimes, they were not always clear. Sometimes, they were complicated, confusing, and difficult on levels that are hard to describe in words. *Pruebas* are spiritual tests.

I remember the first time I heard about *pruebas* during my year long *dieta* in the jungle. A *dieta*, as we have spoken about, is a sacred process of eliminating certain foods, substances, and activities, in order to connect more closely to a master plant, typically a plant chosen by a *curandero* or shaman who holds space for your process. A curandero is a healer or wise medicine person who brings healing and medicine for others. A *dieta* consists of avoiding substances like alcohol, drugs, salt, sugar, red meat, and pork, as well as sexual abstinence, so as to secure the space for a pure connection with the spirit of the master plant.

I had some challenges with forgiving myself for breaking my *dieta* by getting into an argument with one of the facilitators at the center which caused my medicine to turn bad, leaving me feeling sick at the core of my soul for weeks. I wanted to have Ricardo, who was my teacher and *curandero*, clean it; meaning that he would help to dispel the charge of emotions and bring the energies back into alignment. But my facilitator friend was reluctant to put the intentions on the table for this to occur, as it would have made him look bad. So, I had to deal with the issue myself. This issue was that I had crossed my medicine, which at the time, was something I knew nothing about, let alone how to fix it.

Crossing medicine was a new concept to me. Certainly, I had heard the phrase relating to the idea that someone "crossed" me, but I never investigated the term much or took the time to understand the implications of what it really meant. You would think that prior to entering into such a practice like shamanic-medicine work in the jungle, that my shaman would have spoken to me about this. However, I was new to this idea.

The *pruebas* we experience as spiritual tests come in many forms. How one spiritually overcomes and processes any of these hypothetical challenges as they arise in life brings forth the ultimate question: can one maintain a connection to God in such a trying moment? To each and every person, these spiritual tests, or *pruebas,* push our limits and make us either stronger or complacent.

The master shamanic plants are said to help with such spiritual tests, guiding us with their wisdom and knowledge when we, as aspiring shamans or those on the journey of personal healing, connect to them with a willingness to learn and grow. The deeper pressure behind the *prueba* is meant to propel us out of our own karma, to break the inevitable reintroduction of the same pattern that brought us to suffering in the first place. Karma repeats and repeats until it is learned, and we change direction and move closer to the light. The power of the *prueba* is simply that we get to experience a lesson that affects our spiritual strength, and much like any test, the *prueba* comes with reward if we are able to pass it. The reward may be a sense of freedom, joy, or the thrill of new beginnings. If we are not able to pass it, I do not believe that we are punished, like so many shamans I've worked with have asserted, but, rather, that our consciousness is further challenged to discover the truth that we are ultimately the creators of our own existence.

When in your life have you felt that you were being tested by the Universe? Consider the moments when you are confronted with a choice and your mind is unable to construct a quick response. For a simple example, you made a decision to no longer drink alcohol and are actively working through a 12-step program. Your friends invite you to the bar, and you aren't sure what to do. If you're not fully ready to say no to drinking, it could be a slippery slope if you are in the presence of drinking. Should you go or should you stay back and learn to say no, even if it's hard?

A spiritual *prueba* doesn't have a booklet attached to it with the answers that say, "Here's what your lesson is and what to do and what will happen if you don't make the correct choice." Some *pruebas* are harder than others. Some *pruebas* are black and white. The real test is whether you can consciously choose to accept the challenge while maintaining integrity.

We are always being tested. For me, I have come to the belief that the test is not there to push me down, but to help me accelerate into a higher state of consciousness.

It may be helpful to journal about a few times in your life when you had to make a decision that was difficult to make. Perhaps that decision meant you needed to sacrifice something in order to pass through it. Have you learned because of this experience? Or do you find yourself revisiting these *pruebas* over and over again?

No one can go through the *prueba* for you. Just like no one can live your life for you.

CHAPTER 15

The Advocates

The office I worked out of was in downtown San Diego, California. It was owned by a couple who I met while I was studying at the PCOM. I was blessed to be there and grow my practice for several years. The office had a real charm to it, a cozy waiting room, a kitchen with tinctures and herbal granules to make formulas, and a few private rooms to practice my drumming and tobacco work. After I cried into my drum and had all of these miraculous experiences of my life being transformed, I began to ponder new ways I could teach and help others on their own journey.

At the time, I lived in Del Mar with a few friends. The porch out back had a beautiful area for yoga, so I would practice and take breaks and journal ideas. It occurred to me one day that I should offer some services like "ghost-busting", which, I had learned, I was actually pretty good at doing. What I mean by that is simply clearing out spaces that had energy or even spirits lingering around. That was the original idea behind The Advocates. I wanted to create a business that would help people feel comfortable in their own homes and their own skin. I remember growing up in a home that was very obviously haunted, voices from the attic could be heard through the vents, and I always had the feeling that someone was following me everywhere. It was absolutely terrifying to live in such a house as a little girl. Having that traumatic experience, I realized that I could offer people something that I once needed, which was someone advocating for me, so I felt safe and protected in my own home.

The many experiences, both good and bad, I had throughout my life eventually brought me to this path in which The Advocates business began to translate into real solutions to the problems my clients had. It wasn't a business centered around "ghosts"; it had to do with truly caring about the soul of others and the world at large. That is what the world needs right now: people to genuinely care about others and support them along their path, in the same way Kelly did for me.

Could it be possible that she could live on through me as I taught? Could she still be there with me when I worked? I realized over time that this was true. She was there every step of the way. I felt like I was initiating people into this practice or lineage of the "Advocates' way" by sharing that frequency of friendship and love with them, a frequency that helped them purge the energies that were not in resonance with their own being. I felt like I was channeling really beautiful medicine for them, which thus helped them to connect with the true power of their own life force within.

Just like all things in life, there is a beginning, middle, and eventually, an end. In the fall of 2017, after teaching nearly 70 students and initiating about 10 apprentices, I closed the office. I was at the height of my career, but I had to make a very serious decision. I was experiencing sharp, stabbing stomach pain, and it was getting worse and worse. I was having trouble singing and journeying because of it. Although I was still able to help people, I was, nevertheless, suffering from gut-wrenching pain that bothered me on a daily basis. I had enough of leaving the office only to sit in my car and feel this deep sense that something wasn't right. It was my birthday of that year that really illuminated the depth of the despair I was putting myself through. Now, I was making six figures, and I had my doctorate, but I still felt the pain. At one time, I believed having earned a good living and a degree would cure the dis-ease. That was not the case.

On my 30th birthday, I returned home from a ceremony, and I realized I needed to go deeper in my healing path and to commit to the learning and growth necessary if I were to really help people in a more intimate and efficient way. At the time that I made this decision, I had the support of other year-long apprentices I admired, who expressed their support if I needed anything along the way, as they understood the tests that would come once I made the decision to go back to the jungle and complete a year-long shamanic apprenticeship. I was not yet aware of what was to come, but the tests came, and they always come, because I have learned that is how life strengthens our integrity. So, I booked my ticket to Peru to see Ricardo and begin the healing process I needed, yet again. This time, I was not kidding around, so I planned to do the year apprenticeship, so that I could finally unravel what was stuck deep within.

CHAPTER 16

Talking to the Plants

I'm being quarantined
to be quality,
released sometime
in reality.
So that I can see
from a clean lens,
rather than
from suffering.
And so it is.
I'm facing life,
apart from my community
A shaman is birthed
patiently.
No longer will I be
sick with human disease
carried down from generations
of families.
So, I take on this task
of fighting darkness
to see the light,
of knowing truth
amongst false illusions and fear,
so that I may represent
what others know but may question
A strong, noble leader.

—Ashley Tomasino,
Translated wisdom from Ayahuma

To become a shaman—one who carries medicine within their body and wisdom and knowledge in their soul—you must understand the language of the plants. You must understand how vegetative life communicates, and you must be receptive to their energy and their capabilities of language, as they are subtle and very different to human communication. We have been accustomed in our society to drown out the subtleties and less dense interpersonal energies; this graceful and simple energy that plants continually emit to those who have the ears to listen. These energies are powerful and healing, but to actually encounter them, we must change ourselves and heal our traumas, remove blockages, and clear the toxic energies that prevent us from being receptive to their gentle information and guidance.

I believe that all beings in the Universe communicate telepathically. The plants teach us about their wisdom. For instance, they teach us through our dreams by sharing melodies and songs that embody their wisdom which is infused in the melody. Sometimes, they teach us through music, and other times, their universal wisdom is transmitted directly in visions and flashes of intuition during ceremony. We train our consciousness to be open to these messages through practices such as meditation, drumming, or any type of spiritual work that takes us into an altered state of consciousness.

I remember the first time I began talking with the plants. It didn't start with direct plant communication at first; it was talking with animals I encountered during ceremony. When in my first shamanic class, I worked with talking to my first guide, the Lion. He spoke to me telepathically, and I journaled all our conversations on paper, so I would be able to eventually integrate them into my own practice. Learning how to do this and trusting the information I received then translated into my capacity to engage directly with plant consciousness.

Ricardo gave me a diet called Pinon Blanco a few times during my work with him. In 2013, I sat in my tambo after ceremony and meditated in the hammock, alone in the dark. I saw this glowing green light next to me. It was Pinon Blanco. The plant spirit was communicating something to me, so I tuned in with my attention and listened.

"Ashley, if you don't heal your stomach, you will get cancer."

I wrote it down and let it go and didn't think about it for a while, until I was a student at Emperors College of Traditional Chinese Medicine in Santa Monica, California a year later in 2014 and needed an acupuncture treatment session from one of the professors at my school. He told me when he diagnosed my case and palpated my stomach that I would get stomach cancer if I didn't get treatment.

Now, that was a very strong statement to make. I thought to myself, *Shit. What am I going to do?* So, I went back to him to get his opinion again only a few weeks later, and he said he didn't remember saying it at all. I recalled how guides work in mysterious ways and figured either he really forgot, or he was channeling a message from my plants for me. Then, I remembered Pinon Blanco telling me that I needed to work on this.

I sat in another ceremony with the medicine after hearing this news, and as the mareacion$_1$ came on, I saw myself in a hospital bed with beeping monitors and my mother standing over me as I had tubes down my throat. I was about ten years old. The medicine said, "Ashley, you have repressed this memory for so long, but this is at the root of your issues with your stomach."

The medicine knew it was hard for me to look at what it was about to show me. I had to really focus. As I looked, I began to remember the moment when I was in the ER after having just ingesting poisonous cleaning fluid on accident at ten years old. The medicine said that she didn't want me to suffer any longer and that I had to face what had happened. Somehow I had blocked this painful memory out of my mind but my body and soul still remembered and it was at

---

1   Mareacion is the energy of the plant medicine that feels like a natural high. It is when the medicine is said to kick in, where the journeyer who takes the psychedelic plant medicine is most sensitive to the affects it has on their consciousness.

this ceremony that I was shown the truth. The medicine continued to show me this painful scene.

My mother stood over my body and in a terrorizing way said, "Look at what you're doing to me. You're ruining my life!" She stared deeply into my eyes. I looked back at a cold, distant woman and felt like I wanted to die. This was what I thought life was about.

I came out of the scene and back to my mat. I didn't want to go back there. I never wanted to relive that memory from a time when I had no voice or choice in how to protect myself as a kid. I could feel my heart and soul break deeply inside of my body and my craving for a mother was more real and apparent in that moment. I suppose that is why I was attracted to La Madre, the mother of us all—the mother I needed.

I received guidance from my plants after the first few *dietas* with Ricardo, that I should continue my shamanic path. So to engage more deeply with my plants, I decided to develop a system where I went back and forth in conversation with them. The practice then further evolved to recognizing if it was the light of the plant, instead of the dark side of it, that I was actually engaging with. As I learned, there is also what is called *shitana*, which is the dark energy of vegetative life that can be accumulated due to the influence of toxic substances. The language of the plant doesn't always come across as pure medicine, and so shamans learn to differentiate this frequency, so the guidance becomes pure.

I was still dealing with stomach pain for many years into my early 30s that bothered me in every single ceremony. For about probably four hundred ceremonies, I was still struggling with my stomach. You know that old saying, "trust your gut," well, I had such a challenge with that because my stomach lining from the accident with the cleaning fluid and the core of my soul had become sick, due to my many unfortunate childhood experiences and I believe from drinking the poison. So, receiving information was sometimes challenging, because we need to process this information in our gut in order to make decisions regarding the next steps on our journey.

The plants have a unique way of communicating. Sometimes, they can be upfront, and you can literally hear them talking, as if they are on the phone with you. I have found, however, that they speak the most in dreams. They also communicate through melody and song. But however they speak, we can translate their consciousness through our own creative expression. This can occur by focusing on the master plant we are dieting and then playing an instrument, talking to a friend, journaling, or simply contemplating something within. The plants emanate their wisdom, and we can be the receivers of it.

I found that my plants were communicating with me in multiple ways. I remember a ceremony where I saw the Titanic, and my plants were telling me that if I went too fast, just like in Chinese medicine theory, that I would sink. Too much yang, which is fast movement, can lead to excess yin, which can then lead to immobile and freezing cold conditions — or otherwise, death. There must be a balance in the Universe, and the plants were advising me not to go too fast with something.

Ironically, earlier that day, I heard a warning from the plants. The Celine Dion song from *Titanic* was playing on repeat in the office at the center where I completed my year of training. The plants sometimes even communicate to me through Chinese medicine theory because that is the language I understand and comprehend well. That is the medicine I was trained in, so if you're trained as a mathematician or an accountant, the plants will communicate with you through a level of understanding that you can comprehend. Perhaps with synchronicity or through formulas that have meaning to you. They can also communicate through other people as they channel information through to us.

I remember sitting in ceremony once when I asked *Ayahuma* for guidance on what to call my business. I waited and listened. I heard *Ayahuma* say, in a high-pitched Italian-Chicago accent, "The Advocates!"

The Advocates, I thought. It felt right, and it made me think of the feeling I wanted to have when I was growing up, to have an advocate for my own life. I was excited, so I called my dad. He picked up to hear the news. I told him, "Dad! I have the name for my business! Guess what it is?!'

"What is it, Ash?"

"The Advocates!" I said.

"The Advocates?! I like it!" He said in an identical voice-inflection-melody as *Ayahuma,* but as an Italian, 5'6"-tall man with a mustache — and a Chicago accent.

The Advocates then later became the name for my business. I had a dream of developing a system where I helped train shamans to embody the essence of what Kelly gave to me, the feeling of having a real friend who sincerely cared for their lives. This would be my medicine, and through that feeling, I could teach them to journey like I did.

CHAPTER 17

Healing Through the Power
of the Advocate Archetype

Your greatest ally and advocate in life is within you. When I sat in my tambo for nearly two-and-a-half years (on and off through the duration of a seven-year period), I developed a clear sense of the inner Ashley who was my friend and had my best interests in mind. The inner advocate is what my work is meant to help people uncover. Through conscious contact with the wisdom of your own advocate, you can begin to heal and transform wounds and unprocessed emotions. This inner advocate has the tools, the strength, and the awareness to make this happen — as they know your whole story. There is deep and profound compassion in allowing the advocate to have a presence in your life when you sit and let uncomfortable energies arise for the purpose of releasing them.

I remember sitting in my *tambo* one time when I was experiencing a few days of just wanting to complain and say angry things to people I held resentments towards. These were things I didn't feel like journaling, and these were things I didn't want to say to others out loud. Instead, I let myself just listen to what the inner dialogue had to say. Simply by hearing myself out, I gave myself permission to express the frustrations and truth that I really felt about things. My inner advocate was there for me and understood my hurt and frustration. Often, when we want to share anger or frustrations, it seems that our society is conditioned to want to fix it, block, or change the narrative about why we are hurt, and why that anger is even coming up in the first place.

What the pain needs is a space to share without interference. The advocate within us is an awareness or energy that can properly address the concerns and anger we have and then witness its expression. The inner advocate does not need to change you; it doesn't take what you're saying personally, and it knows how valuable the process of speaking what is true within can be for your health.

When the body resists this expression, it has been scientifically proven that these emotions are stored in the cellular field of the body and can even result in disease. To heal yourself, I suggest calling in your inner-advocate and exposing your soul to that consciousness that can assess and properly address those concerns that have left you feeling blocked.

In Chinese medicine, when the energies are blocked, we call this *Qi stagnation*. Usually, this Qi stagnation is related to the liver. The liver is correlated to the emotion of anger or resentment that has not been processed. To move this anger, we use acupuncture points like Liver 3 on the foot or Ren 6 below the umbilicus. If you are in ceremony or in a *dieta* and you're feeling like you cannot access the wisdom of the advocate, something simple you can do is to massage the point between your big toe and second toe. You may even feel a dull, achy sensation when you do this. You can do this for a few minutes, or until you feel you have made a change in the energy and can clearly speak about what is upsetting you.

In Shipibo shamanism, we sing:

sinatai ochabo,
jawen ocha yabi menenquin
sina ina tai ochabo
chodo chodo vainquin.

This means, "The *ocha* from your anger, I gather all the *ocha* of anger, and I clear, and I'm clearing this energy." *Ocha* is anger in Shipibo. *Ocha* is a term used to describe the particular frequency of energy related to the emotions of guilt, shame, fear, or any energy related to that core emotion of anger.

So, for example, the shaman may sing *icaros* for establishing a directness of understanding that there is, in fact, *ocha*. Calling it out by its name and then gathering it and sending it to the light or to be burned, can relieve the charge from these energies:

ocha ocha yamebo
mesko ocha kanobo
tsinki tsinki vainquin
jawen ocha yabe menenquin.
menen menen vainquin

The shaman can sing these *icaros*, but what is more important is that the strength, the melody, and the intention match the particular frequency of the energy that is coming up to be processed.

One thing I've learned about *ocha* is that everyone has ocha around something that has happened in their lives. Perhaps it's *ocha* around an experience that has left you feeling guilt or shame. As Ricardo would say, just clean the *ocha*, no matter where it came from.

I liked his approach, because he emphasized not getting into the story, which is often what keeps us attached and, in a way, even empowers the *ocha* to continue blocking us in our lives.

Keep it simple. If you feel the *ocha*, you can address it with various techniques that I've described above. Certainly, there are unique qualities based on the situation, but I like Ricardo's approach especially because when we get lost in the story, we miss out on connection to the medicine that the *prueba* was there to help us with. Clearing the anger is an important piece if it arises. And, in accessing the archetype of the advocate, which is essentially pure love and understanding, we can then have more space to be aware of the energies that are stuck and causing disharmony in our lives.

There is a pattern in Chinese medicine called "liver overacting on the stomach." Sometimes, people have stomach problems because the liver attacks the energy of the stomach. If you're feeling sick to your stomach after being upset, this may be the cause. I know from growing up that when I held emotions in, I couldn't eat and had stomach pain. Today, I see this a lot with my patients. The typical protocol in dealing with this from a Chinese medicine perspective is to first course the liver energy by moving the Qi, which is a term used to describe energy in the body, and then strengthen the Qi of the stomach. There may also be purging involved, which can help remove the toxic energies from unprocessed emotions that interfere with the stomach.

The stomach, as the second brain of our body, is also part of our processing center. We psychologically process events in our life through our consciousness and through our inner wisdom located in our gut. When the liver attacks the stomach, the second brain of the body is compromised.

Coming back to the archetype of the advocate, it's important to remember that you are your own best healer and doctor, *so trust your gut.* If you feel you need to get healing and something is brewing from the result of not addressing old pain, do something to address this. Remember that your best advocate is the one inside. Learning how to discern the voice of the advocate can be a little challenging at first, but keep listening, and eventually, the voice will be crystal clear. This friend wants the best for you and loves you unconditionally. The inner advocate can be channeled anytime you need him/her. You can also practice asking your inner advocate for help or to understand the five questions. See what they say and practice journaling, so you can integrate this powerful consciousness.

CHAPTER 18

Applying the Five Questions

The five questions that were first asked by the child in the hospital, and then on the beach by the group of teenagers, were not just applicable during my own healing experience, but I also found them to be medicine in random moments of stress, anxiety, or any other unpleasant emotional experiences for others that tested my ability to stay present to witness their experiences. The first question, "What is the meaning of life," and my answer "to have an experience," automatically puts me in the seat of the observer in simply witnessing my life from a bird's eye view. This experience of detachment allows for the meditative and healing space to open.

When in your life have you felt like the world has come crashing down, leaving you feeling helpless or hopeless, perhaps like a victim? These emotionally distressing experiences can leave us feeling like no amount of consoling from friends can ease the discontentment we feel at the soul level. The first question asks, essentially, are you awake and aware to the experience that you are having as a soul in a human body? And more importantly, can you not take this experience personally, even if it is difficult, enough to accept that it is simply an experience?

I can tell when one of my students gets lost in their story. It's like their eyes glaze over, and the situation they're suffering through is a direct reflection of their worth, challenging their inner narrative about what they believe their life is about. They are disconnected from the present moment, from their breath, and from the power of their essence and truth. We have all experienced this before. It's that moment when something traumatic happens and we lose sense of our, well, senses! It's the moment when the only question to ask is, what is the meaning of life, and then knowing that you are right here, right now having an experience as a soul traveling in your human body. The difficult circumstances you may be in currently, or have been in before, are moments that have helped define your character, to grow, and to evolve into a more complete human being and enlightened soul.

This understanding that we are having an experience takes away from any narrative about the *why* and *how*. Why me? Why this? Why now? How could he? How is this possible?

In the moment, when we're asking yourself what the meaning of life is, there is no why question involved, because the simple truth takes away the charge related to any emotion related to the victim. The question, itself, sets the tone for our sane, rational self to come into focus and to understand the simplicity of being.

You can start with noticing your thoughts as you sit and have tea or coffee in the morning and say to yourself, "I am having an experience. I am experiencing the taste of this coffee. I am experiencing my body feeling at ease in this chair as I read the news." Taking the moment into focus allows for the divine, natural flow to enter your stream of consciousness as it softens the mood, turns down the noise, and gets right to the truth of your reality. There is nothing more to think about, and *you have then left the space open for God to enter.*

How does God enter our lives? I believe God is already in our life. Everywhere we go, whatever we do, or whatever circumstances, God is with us. By being receptive to this moment, we allow the space for God to enter and bless us with his presence, the presence of love.

And as to the second question, "Do you believe in God?"

I remember being about two or three years old when my family would go to church on Sunday morning to listen to Pastor Chuck speak his sermon. I was confused about who God was, because Pastor Chuck talked about him like he was actually a living human being. Who is this amazing person who loves everyone and forgives so easily? One day, I went up to Pastor Chuck and asked him, "Are *you* God?"

He chuckled and said, "No, Ashley, I'm not God, but God is within you!"

After I recalled that experience on the podium, I believed in God and understood that I could connect to this loving presence through consciously meditating on the memory of that day when I was a little girl. I don't believe we have to even believe in a formal religious sense that God exists for God to be with us, because that seems more like a human need for validation than a genuine spiritual encounter.

Have you ever noticed that by contemplating God, you just feel better? Have you prayed to God for a miracle and then something beyond what you had expected occurs?

I was speaking with a friend recently about believing in God. We agreed that God is always present, but it is up to us to stay present and know deep within that we are not alone. I have to remind myself that even when life gets dark and frightening, and seems like anything *but* heaven, that even in those dark places, God is still with me. The saying, *As I walk through the valley of the shadow of death, I will fear no evil, for thine is with me, thy rod and thy staff comfort me*, applies.

During that conversation, I was reminded of the time when I saw Kelly in my visions during an ayahuasca ceremony and she was standing near her grave, saying she was scared to go to the other side. I told her that even if she were in hell, that I would go there and bring her to the light, that she was not alone. The feeling that came through me was pure love, the type of advocacy for her soul that I train my students and apprentices to understand that I learned from her. It's the type of love that is solid through thick and thin, heaven or hell, because that love is the essence of the strength of the Creator, Himself. Without fear and without doubt, that essence can transcend any level of the perils of the human condition. It was through loving her as such a dear friend that I came to know what and who God was to me, and I feel grateful for that.

In what ways have others shown up for you with righteous passion to stand up for your soul? This is an important question, because I believe we all need real friends who genuinely care. When we feel connected to others who understand us and feel us on this deep level, we do not feel the despair of loneliness. That advocacy for our own soul can heal the loneliness within and help to cure the co-dependency we may feel towards others, because what we seek outside is purely within (if loneliness and codependency is what you're dealing with). To be our own best friend is the doorway to the kingdom of heaven, the freedom to be understood and cared for, even when we are sick, lost, or alone, and most certainly felt without judgment.

The third question is, "Do you believe God has a plan for you?" God's plan for you is to love yourself, and as the plan may be written in the stars, we are still active participants with free will. I have come to learn that destiny is not something anyone can tell me will or will not happen. Destiny is the unfolding of events as they are in this moment and through the momentum of previous experiences. If I believe God had a plan for me, it would be to live my life embracing healthy love, creating beautiful works of art, sharing my heart, and learning more about what life is about. When I've attached myself to what I think God's plan is for me, I set myself up for disappointment, because I don't know what those specifics are, even though I've tried to write it out in detail. I don't believe that God's plan is for me to do destructive things or choose fear over joy. God is a co-creator and I like sharing with Him about what I would like to have and experience, and I feel that we work together to make those things manifest in my waking reality.

Perhaps if you'd like to try talking to God, not just through prayer, but actively having a conversation, you can journal back and forth, starting with your non-dominant hand, as if it were the inner child, and your dominant hand representing the God force conversing with your inner child. I like to do this exercise and feel into the essence of my higher self, who is speaking lovingly with me about whatever it is my heart desires to have a conversation about. This practice builds the bond within and helps to identify what thoughts or feelings may not be loving and to discern between them more clearly. You can try doing this by writing:

Little Ashley: *Hi, I'm little Ashley, and I'd like to talk with you. Will you talk to me?*

God/Higher Self: *Hi, little Ashley, I would love to talk with you. What would you like to talk about?*

Once you establish a connection, the conversation should move smoothly. You may find a great amount of healing through this practice and notice how much better you feel about your situation.

If things have not turned out as you had planned, it's important to remember that God always pulls you back on track, with enough patience and courage to be your best advocate, that love will always be there for you to lean back on and recreate a new and even better plan full of the love and joy you seek and very much deserve.

The fourth question is, "Do you believe God loves you? The short answer is *yes*. Of course, God loves you and all things in the Universe, because that is what God is. God has no other agenda but to be exactly it. God does not have human qualities nor judge us, because the loving presence that God is only functions to shine the light on our essence, which is pure and beautiful, real and divine.

If you are in the presence of those who you don't feel loved by, perhaps you might be picking up on their energy. Perhaps they don't practice self-love, or they don't accept themselves fully. In their presence, you may feel blocked or limited and take it personally. It's important to remember that turning back to the connection with God as you see or feel Him will allow for that presence to enter more fully.

In the beginning of my shamanic practice with Mary Kay, I wanted to connect with loving guides like my lion. Throughout my relationship with this lion, I felt more accepted and adored than ever before in my life. When people were hurtful towards me or said mean things, I would brush it off and think to myself, "Would my lion ever say that to me?" The answer was no, most definitely not. Our guides, angels, and best teachers do not have the ability to act in ways that are harmful to our souls. If you sense this when you connect to what you feel is God, then that is not God at all. God is pure love, and it's important to always remember that, as well as remembering that humans are humans, we have faults and flaws, and we are not perfect. People are doing their best, even if we see them as not doing their best. When we know deeply within that God loves us, there is a real strength and freedom to be sovereign and walk on the planet with an advocate by our side.

"What happens when we die?"

Certainly, this last question is not something that I can say for certain, because I am still living and breathing. Those who have experienced near death experiences—or NDEs—share about their journey to the light and back. Some have profound experiences of being in an alternate, blissful universe, where they are met by angels and loved ones who have passed. The beauty that I hear about gives me hope that this isn't all there is to my existence as Ashley. I want to know that Ashley deserves a place in the divine realms to continue embracing her essence. I speak in third person, because my perspective changes when I observe what would happen if I lifted off into another realm.

The Egyptians believed in an afterlife, prepping their corpses for the next journey ahead. Many ancient societies believed this and would adorn their loved ones with gifts and jewelry and even money for their next voyage out of this world.

The question was significant to me at the time it was asked, because in the moment of great despair and wishing I were dead so the pain would end, I hadn't considered, what would happen if I actually *did* die? In the moment when everything seems so emotionally hurtful and stressful that you want to give up on life, who is to say that hurting yourself and taking your own life will lead you to a better and happier place? The gamble is not worth taking, even though things can get bad here. Taking the time to breathe through it, finding the courage to ask for help, waiting at least a week until things pass — all seem like torture. The pain can be so overwhelming that living another day feels like punishment.

Even though I've had amazing experiences with God and have come to a place of trusting that God is with me always, that I am loved, and that my life has purpose, I am reminded of the fact that this is just an experience, and that even this experience will change. Life is impermanent, everything changes, nothing stays the same, and nothing is forever, except love. Love transcends time and space because it is that powerful.

When I die, I pray that I meet my loved ones in heaven and that my soul can continue living as the beautiful being I saw in the light of the reflection of God. The journey of life makes chapters end and then begin again, and the pages turn and become like books on shelves in the record of life. These pieces of experiences we are having, albeit some incredible or sad, will forever be imprinted in the book of our life. As the main character, you get to choose how you move through the obstacles and challenges of the soul's path. The death piece may also come as the shedding of old skins, the new awakening of a life worth being born into or walking a path that you have never walked before.

CHAPTER 19

The Dark Night of the Soul

After having a conversation with one of my *maestros*, I wanted to understand the hero's journey, a process laid out in a book by the American writer Joseph Campbell, even more. In the book, he talks about the experience of going through an initiation process that inevitably brings us to a new path through the darkness of uncertainty and challenges that we would have otherwise never experienced. It is through our own hero's journey that we are tested and challenged to face the inner demons within and to find the strength to trust our divine gifts through embracing the path ahead. After going through the cycle of the hero's journey, we are never the same, and more importantly, can never return to the place we once were before embarking on this journey — *that is the whole point.*

The dark night of the soul is just one chapter in the book of your hero's journey and encompasses the *pruebas* necessary to learn what is essential for the evolution of your hero's path and your soul.

A journey will never be all love and light and sunshine and unicorns with rainbows with gold at the end. It will never be all that, because that is not the way life works. Nature works in cycles. The dark night, although it can seem scary to think of entering a darkness, as we are trained to believe that black means bad and darkness means evil, is the yin essence, just like the yang is the daytime. Each day, the sun sets, and we see the moon in the sky. The darkness of night does not necessarily mean all is literally dark. It just means we are walking through a shadow. This shadow is essential to our understanding of all the facets of what it means to be a whole and integrated human being.

I remember each night after ceremony would end or after I received my song from the shaman who sang to me, I would depart the *maloca* and return to my *tambo*. Or sometimes, I would walk far into the jungle while still under the effect of the ayahuasca *mariacion*. Sometimes, I felt uncomfortable walking alone at night through the forest, and I would begin to sing or say the prayer, *"As I walk through the valley of the shadow of death, I fear no evil, for thine is with me, thy rod and thy staff comfort me."*

There is no stronger level of courage than to feel the power of God walking beside you, even if you're walking through hell. In my experiences of going through the dark night of the soul, I eventually discovered that it was just a walk and that I had to keep moving forward, *no matter what happened next.* A common phrase is, "If you're in hell, keep going." There is no need to stay trapped in the dark night. We must understand we are involved in a process, a process that will culminate in becoming a new person, a regenerated and renewed human being.

The dark night is not something you can call upon yourself at will, as I believe it is a spontaneous encounter. When I say encounter, I mean something that is thrust upon us without our consent. No matter how bad it may appear, if you understand that what you're going through is a process of initiation and development, you will always come out empowered. And you will eventually be able to hold your own staff or sword with the type of humility and honor that no one can ever take away from you. The complete release of the ego from being humbled by the yin of the night of your soul will soften the sharpness of anger, it will open your heart to compassion, and it will allow you to see your true humanity.

Ultimately, it will allow you to feel the deep, internal strength of your inner advocate, who is there for you through the thickness of confusion, fear, and suffering. There is no love like the love of a friend who has your back unconditionally.

If your dark night is happening right now, I encourage you to practice working with the five questions. Let the answers carry you deeper into your own true wisdom and knowledge within. This is the yin essence, the divine feminine essence that contains the life-force of the subconscious world. Let the questions carry you along to find the true answers that define your purpose. There is no greater teacher than the dark, no greater witness than the life-force within, and no greater humbling power than facing head on; our shadow.

Letting the past go, not trying to change in our minds what should have been or what could have been, is part of facing what the dark night is meant to teach us. No one dwells on the past who is content with the moment. It is only when we are not accepting of reality that we wish things could have been different. I, myself, went through hell, but I kept going. I kept living, and I never gave up on myself. The inner advocate always lives within us and will continue to walk with us, whether we are in the light or in the dark. This is what I stand for with my friends, loved ones, and patients. No matter what, we must stand strong and tall for each other, to hold the light of divine reflection.

I believe the dark night of the soul was a profound experience that has shaped my sense of compassion, empathy, and acceptance of others. It has provided the contrast to see when people are talking to me who are inauthentic or not very integrated.

It was the dark night that I always feared, because I didn't know if I could make it out alive. Would I lose everything I loved? Would I fall apart and actually die?

What happened was…*I found myself.*

CHAPTER 20

The Path of Love

It was 2015, and I decided to bring a group to see Ricardo. We arrived, and I could tell this trip would be a unique one, namely because there's a feeling that we all get when we approach La Madre. It's auspicious, and it feels like a pull to ceremony. I arrived with the intention of deeper healing because I had some pain in my liver that I couldn't clear on my own. I was in the hospital with an unknown etiology that the medical doctors couldn't figure out the cause of.

I had crippling physical pain that kept me hospitalized for four days, ironically in the oncology department in San Diego. After running some tests, the doctors determined there was nothing wrong and discharged me. I called a friend who works in the shamanic field to look. He said he saw something dark, like a snake, blocking my liver. I immediately knew I had to take another trip to Ricardo to see what it was. In Chinese medicine, the liver has to do with being able to move forward in life and seeing the path ahead.

When I arrived with my group, I was feeling the crippling pain on my side, but I could still function and walk around without falling over. I shared this with Ricardo, and so, he gave me Tammamuri-bota. Tammamuri is one of my favorite trees to diet, because it has to do with time travel, the wisdom of the womb, and healing trauma.

During one ceremony, I could feel the liver begin to cramp and send waves of shock throughout my body. I rolled around on the mat in agony that began disturbing those around me. As the medicine began to take effect, I called out to Benoit, the helper in ceremony. It was hard to breathe, and I felt delirious. I wanted to run out of my body that felt like it was dying from the inside out.

He came to me and tried to help me as I crawled to the bathroom. I felt like a baby, but weak and heavy, as if the Earth was pulling me towards her to die. I couldn't make it back to my mat without him carrying me there. As he reached down to pick me up, the force of the energies from the Earth pulled me to her and he struggled to lift my 120-pound body up. When he finally did and placed me back on my mat, he began to palpate my body to help me settle down. My visions began to open, and I saw the most beautiful vision I had ever seen in my life.

I didn't know what the Kene was, even after all the years I had been working with the medicine at that point. The Kene are the lines in the medicine you see also on tapestries that the shamans weave, which represent the dimensions of the songs. When the shaman sings, they may see the Kene and use it to help them diagnose the patient. The Kene is the destiny map that emanates outward from the core of our soul. It's most typically seen in our solar plexus, but in this vision, I saw as I lay on my mat in agony, the Kene was overlaying the stars in the sky in the background, where my daughter in the vision lay in her cradle on a windowsill. I could see her face so clearly. Her body was calm and restful, and I could hear the waves in the ocean below. I had asked the medicine how I could ever have this, and I heard her say, "*You have to do the year.*"

Tammamuri helped me calm my senses and see what was deep within me. Although I do not have children now, what I needed to see was that my dream of being a mother could come true. I asked the medicine what her name was and heard clearly, "Lilly."

I immediately fell in love.

When I saw this vision, it resonated on every cell of my body, and my liver stopped cramping. I felt deeply at peace, and I knew it was more than just a vision; it was my medicine.

Although the man who I saw would be the father of Lilly is now married and has a child with his wife, I know the medicine gave me this vision, because I needed to believe that I was worthy of my dreams coming true, and this gave me the courage to enter my year, with the bravery to try becoming the woman who would be her mother. This gave me the strength to fight and commit to isolation for that time alone in the jungle. Everything I fought for was for this beautiful dream. I wonder every day, had I not crossed my diet, if that dream would have become a reality. Such is the way of Zen, to accept what is currently in my reality. Now, I am living my life after my diet, and I am learning how to accept, grow, and continue forward.

The path of love is the path of finding the inner relationship to our highest self, our own advocate. When I wanted to quit, I would go back to the five questions; I would remember these energies and connect to them. I realized that life will always give me spiritual *pruebas* to test the strength of my faith and my medicine, and that my job is to forgive myself when I make mistakes, because I am human, and I have faults, by default! The practice of being enlightened seems to simply be the practice of aligning myself with my dreams and trusting the process as it unfolds.

If the path of love asks you to become a painter, a musician, a mother, or a writer, that is the divine path of shamanic awakening. Becoming a *curandero* is not the only way to walk this path. Everyone who is on their journey of love will inevitably be tested, go through a cycle, and with the guidance from a higher power, eventually be aligned with their higher self, a state of being that may be beyond what they could ever dream. I never dreamed that I would be where I am today, and it was through surrendering to what was deep within my heart, asking for healing and guidance, that I have been blessed with this current reality and ability to share with honesty, integrity, humility, and sincere care for others what I have been through.

In certain moments, we might not be able to see the potential gold that awaits us further along in the journey. However, it is my prayer and belief that upon reviewing the events that have unfolded in our own lives, we can be given the most powerful gift — to be a witness to the life force coming through us and to embrace the power of love. Regardless of past mistakes or difficult learning experiences, love always finds a way.

On my own path, there have always been helpers and kind souls who could see me when I could not see myself and friends who stood with me in solidarity. There was always the miracle of new beginnings, discovering higher perspectives, and profound transformations. I hope for all people to experience this.

There are no trophies, there is only the question: *Are you connected to love in this Zen moment of now?* Perhaps, even if you are struggling to remember, or have fallen off your path, your higher self knows and sends angels your way to help remind you. At least, I would like to think so.

It is my prayer that all people can sense their divine wisdom within. Somehow, that between Zen, the moment of oneness and peace, and now, this experience in the present moment, we can align with the best version of ourselves that we are meant to become.

Amen.

ACKNOWLEDGEMENTS

I would like to acknowledge the people who have inspired my work over the years, those who have made an impression on my soul and who have helped guide my path forward.

First, I would like to acknowledge my Shipibo Maestro, Ricardo Amaringo for fighting for my soul, encouraging me to be the best ayahuasquera I can be, and for all the years he helped me grow. Dr. Daniel Domoleczny, my cousin and friend, for being a comrade on the journey of healing and learning. Thank you for always being there for me and encouraging me and cheering me on. You are a blessing in my life. My dad, my first advocate on the healing journey. Your words of wisdom, encouragement, and support are golden. My sisters, Lisa and Kim, both of you are such an inspiration in your own unique ways. Your spirits were with me every step of the way during my training. I love you both. Thank you for that. My beloved Uncle Joe, you live forever in my heart as my first inspiration to the healing path and as a guide on this journey. Thank you for your light and guidance when I was a little one. I could not have become the woman I am today without you. My Mom, because without you, I would never have had the impetus to heal and fight for my soul.

Dr. East Harradin, DAOM, LAc, thank you for your guidance and passionate encouragement to finally make this dream of publishing my book a reality. I have great admiration for your work and presence in our TCM community. You are a gift to me, and I am so grateful for how you show up for others and myself at such a pivotal time.

Eti Domb LAc, a wonderful healer and businesswoman who I was so blessed to share an office space with for many years. Thank you for the opportunity and the space to grow. Richard Grossman, OMD, Z'ev Rosenberg, LAc, I have great respect for you and your support during the most important moments of my career. Thank you for all you helped me unravel and evolve from to be the practitioner I am today. Allison Snowden, DAOM, LAc, you are such an incredible friend and gift in my life. I have so much gratitude for you sharing this path with me. Russell Feingold, thank you for being an inspiration with your heartfelt dedication to your path, your book, your practice, and your wisdom. You were one of the earliest pioneers in my dieting world, and I would not have done the "year" if I hadn't met you. I have always admired you. Joe Tafur, MD, what words can describe the lessons I've learned from you? You were always such an inspiration to me. Thank you for the gifts you gave me that supported me in my journey of healing. Benoit Allouche, thank you for your efforts to support me in being the best ayahuasquera I could be, for standing up for me and sharing your wisdom and insight. You inspired me to be stronger, healthier, and sing from my soul. You were there for the most powerful and crucial moments of my development, and I couldn't have asked for a more perfect person to witness this. Thank you to Michael Sonn, my friend and maestro. You helped me through so much from the moment we first talked. I can't imagine where I'd be without you since the journey of integration started. I am truly blessed to have met you and call you a friend. Thank you so much.

Shout out to acknowledge my comrades who have loved me on this journey, Drew Taylor, Erin Ward, Emily Sturgeon, Nate Heidi,

Najah Abdus Salaam, Simone Ressner, Marina S., Kenneth Miller, Jonathan Lenahan, Melissa Creamer, David Hatfield, David Ben-Chetrit, Daniel Miller, and Bridgett Shrank.

Ellen Katz, thank you for all you held space for in such a loving, nurturing, and kind way. I am very grateful for all the work you did with me and the healing practice you shared with me for so many years. Ron and Loretta Larson, thank you for being so supportive and believing in me, for accepting me like family, and for encouraging me to write this book. I am so grateful to you for helping me believe in myself, too. Sheryl Stern, my financial advisor, where in the world would I be without you?—dear lord! You are more than just an advisor, but a trusted friend. Bless your heart forever. Nick Rios, a trusted confidant and healer, your alliance on this path is such a blessing, thank you. Gina Tang, your magnificent appearance at the most miraculous moments of my career and my personal life have inspired me to really dive into the work for the business of The Advocates and the beginning stages of really believing in this book. Your work with me was priceless, and I am deeply grateful for our time and work together. This would never have come to fruition in such a way without your guidance and support, love, and friendship. Thank you so much, Gina.

Anna Calisto and Thonger, Wiler, and those who were there for me when I returned back to the world after my year. Your love and support is truly admirable. Thank you for showing up for me and for the work you are doing for the world and for yourself!

My supportive therapist, Marlon Guarino. What a sincere blessing of divine luck that I found you of all the people in the world. I don't know where I'd be without you. Thank you for the work you are doing.

Lizette Rodriguez, Modern Medicine Woman, my first shaman, my spiritual mother and friend…I am blessed to have you in my life as my mentor all these years. So much love to you.

To all my trusted clients, apprentices, students, and acupuncture patients, thank you for believing in me and trusting me to support you. You gave life to my work and helped me integrate through witnessing your powerful journeys. You know who you are!

Francine Duffy and Patrick Duffy, thank you for your trust and faith in me and helping me get going in the early days of my work. You are such a blessing. Alan James, my neighbor and muse. You know what I'd say.

Thank you to all my friends from LZHS, PCOM, ECTOM, NUHS, CIIS, and NIU, what a blessed life to have you to share this journey with. You know who you are!

I'd like to acknowledge Krikor Andonian, PhD. I had you in mind when I wrote this book, as if I was confessing my truth to you, which helped me to finally pull it together after 12 years of work. Ever since we met, I've been in such admiration for you and your passion on your journey.

I'd like to acknowledge the inspiring shamans and thought leaders who helped me see the light through the darkness, whether it be through our connection or their inspirational books and offerings I have read over the years; Alberto Villoldo, Don Miguel Ruiz and Don Miguel Ruiz Jr., Sandra Ingerman, Edgar Cayce, Michael Newton, Bia Labate, the founder of Chacruna and author of several books, articles, and speeches about psychedelics, Rick Doblin, the founder of MAPS, Jen Sincero, Megan Rapinoe, Quinn-the first trans, non binary Olympic soccer player who is such an inspiration.

I'd like to thank the master plants. The powerful, healing plants that have blessed my path all these years; Ayahuma, Tammamuri-

Abota, Pinon Blanco, Ajo Sacha, Chiric Sanango, Tobacco, Nihue Rao, Bombinsana, Coca, and Oje. Of course, also, La Madresita Ayahuasquita. With humble gratitude, I bow to the love and healing from the plants that have blessed my life so deeply. You are my allies, and I am forever humbled by your gifting me and seeing me through to the light.

Last, but certainly not least. Thank you, Kelly Gatsakos. I dedicated this book to you, because without you, I would never have known a love so deep and so profound that would put me on my knees in such a way that I would have the courage to take this journey where it has gone. What words can describe how important, meaningful, and divine it was to be part of your life, to have experienced your friendship, to have been blessed with having such a dear and kind friend like you. You have given me more than I could ever ask for. I am forever honored and humbled by the gift that God has given me—the blessing of someone to share such meaningful time with and that we were able to connect in this lifetime. I hope the essence of this book and the magnitude of my gratitude reaches your soul, wherever you are, and that you feel my love that is eternal. I hope you know just how many lives you've touched through your presence in my practice, that you are deeply missed, and how much you mattered to me and so many others. May you fly higher than mountaintops, so high that the wind won't stop you. And may you rest forever in sweet peace, my dearest friend.

FOR THE READER

This book was written with great honor and perseverance from over 12 years of hard work and dedication. It has taken many iterations and edits to finally feel like I was ready to send off into the world. It started with a painful event of loss and suffering, then it turned out to be quite a beautiful story. Because of the love I experienced, I was able to know how to feel deeply the events I went through to get here. This book is for those who have a soul, who have felt lost or alone in their lives, who have felt like they had no reason to live or struggled to find the courage to be authentically who they are. After all I've endured, I would say honestly that I believe I have something to live for and that feels really wonderful. I hope that all people feel they have something to live for and the questions help define the trajectory of the purpose of their lives, of your life and of the life of your soul for eternity.

Thank you for reading my book. I wrote it for you, with love, and I hope you can feel me and my intention to support you to being the best version of yourself, wherever you are currently and wherever you are going. My intention is that this book may accompany you on your journey, and that you can have it with you if and when you need it, like a light in the dark. My ultimate message and hope for you is; *May you always feel you have an advocate and friend with you, between Zen and now.*

ABOUT THE AUTHOR

Dr. Ashley Tomasino is a board certified and licensed acupuncturist and herbalist in California. She has completed extensive training in her internships by working at Rady Children's Hospital, Warren's HIV Clinic in San Diego, California, and studying under masters of ayahuasca shamanism. She has trained with master teachers, such as Mary Kay Ryan in the Michael Harner Foundation way. She has a doctorate in Chinese medicine from Emperor's College of Traditional Chinese Medicine. She also holds a master's degree in acupuncture and Chinese medicine from Pacific College of Oriental Medicine and a bachelor's degree in biomedical science from National University of Health Sciences. After creating a successful medical practice, she decided to pursue entering a formal apprenticeship by working with master plants in isolation, which counted for a cumulative total of two-and-a-half years with Maestro Ricardo Amaringo, an Onaya Shipibo Ayahuasquero in Iquitos, Peru, in order to learn the traditional way to hold ceremonies, to heal, and to master the songs; icaros.. Dr Ashley was the youngest apprentice to undergo the rigorous one year of isolation apprenticeship under Ricardo's tutelage. She has founded The Advocates Institute for Shamanic Studies, Inc. Dr. Ashley has trained countless apprentices to learn her methods and techniques for spiritual healing using the integration of Chinese medicine, core shamanism and ayahuasca shamanism. Dr. Ashley is currently a doctoral student at California Institute of Integral Studies to achieve her second PhD in philosophy.

To connect with Dr. Ashley, you can visit www.DrAshleyTomasino.org.